ALSO BY DAVID B. AGUS, MD

The End of Illness

A SHORT GUIDE TO A LONG LIFE

—

DAVID B. AGUS, MD
with Kristin Loberg

Illustrations by Chieun Ko-Bistrong

SIMON & SCHUSTER
New York   London   Toronto   Sydney   New Delhi

Simon & Schuster
1230 Avenue of the Americas
New York, NY 10020

Text copyright © 2014 by Dr. David B. Agus
Illustrations © 2014 by Chieun Ko-Bistrong

First Simon & Schuster hardcover edition January 2014

SIMON & SCHUSTER and colophon are
registered trademarks of Simon & Schuster, Inc.

For information about special discounts for bulk purchases, please contact Simon & Schuster Special Sales at 1-866-506-1949 or business@simonandschuster.com.

The Simon & Schuster Speakers Bureau can bring authors to your live event. For more information or to book an event contact the Simon & Schuster Speakers Bureau at 1-866-248-3049 or visit our website at www.simonspeakers.com.

Designed by Nancy Singer

Manufactured in the United States of America

10 9 8 7 6 5 4 3 2 1

Library of Congress Cataloging-in-Publication Data

Agus, David, 1965–
A short guide to a long life / David B. Agus, MD., with Kristin Loberg ; illustrations by Chieun Ko-Bistrong. — First Simon & Schuster hardcover edition.
    pages cm
1. Longevity. 2. Aging—Nutritional aspects. 3. Physical fitness. 4. Self-care, Health.
    I. Loberg, Kristin. II. Title.
    RA776.75.A38 2014
    613.2—dc23   2013024329
    ISBN 978-1-4767-3095-0
    ISBN 978-1-4767-3096-7 (ebook)

To my wife, partner, and love,
Amy Povich,
and our genetic experiments gone right,
Sydney and Miles

A BRIEF HISTORICAL NOTE

Hippocrates was a Greek physician in the time of the third and fourth century BC. Modern medicine refers to Hippocrates as the father of Western medicine. He was among the first physicians to convey important "health rules" through his many now-famous quotes. Below are some examples that continue to have amazing relevance to today's medicine. In fact, one could argue that our modern world has brought science and data into the field, but his initial observations and recommendations were remarkably accurate over two thousand years ago.

Walking is man's best medicine.

Let food be thy medicine and medicine be thy food.

Declare the past, diagnose the present, foretell the future.

Primum non nocerum. (First, do no harm.)

It is far more important to know what person the disease has than what disease the person has.

If we could give every individual the right amount of nourishment and exercise, not too little and not too much, we would have found the safest way to health.

A wise man should consider that health is the greatest of human blessings, and learn how by his own thought to derive benefit from his illnesses.

Everything in excess is opposed to nature.

To do nothing is also a good remedy.

There are in fact two things, science and opinion; the former begets knowledge, the latter ignorance.

Hippocrates (c. 460 BC–c. 370 BC)

CONTENTS

A SHORT GUIDE
TO A LONG LIFE

Introduction: The Power of Prevention

At least twice a week, I tell a patient that I have nothing left in my arsenal to combat his or her cancer. It's over, and in most cases the end is near. I've never gotten used to this gut-wrenching conversation. But I do it as part of the role I've accepted. That we are no better at treating cancer today, with a few notable exceptions, than we were fifty years ago is maddening. More infuriating still is that many of my patients could have prevented their cancer or other life-altering disease had they done a few things differently earlier in life. That makes those conversations even more upsetting. I'm pretty certain that most people could delay or totally prevent a vast majority of the illnesses we see today—including not only cancer but heart and kidney disease, stroke, obesity, diabetes, autoimmune disorders, and dementia and other neurodegenerative disorders—if they just adopt a few healthy habits early on and avoid the ones that lead to illness.

The best way to fight not just cancer but all the other ailments that typically develop over time is to prevent them. A staggering seven out of ten deaths among Americans each year are from chronic diseases like the ones I just named. Heart disease, cancer, and stroke account for more than 50 percent of all deaths every year. About half of us are living with a chronic condition right now.

But prevention is a hard sell. Think about yourself for a moment: can you see yourself twenty, thirty, or forty years from now? We all want to live however we choose today and pay our dues later. I see this payment being made by my patients daily, just by looking into their eyes.

I'd like nothing more than to be put out of my job. Imagine a world where we all die of old age—our bodies go kaput, much like an old car with hundreds of thousands of great miles on it. One day, the engine doesn't start and nothing can revive it. In fact, 1951 was the last year you could die in the United States with the cause "old age" being listed on the death certificate. Since then, we've had to name a specific disease, injury, or complication. I find it astonishing to think that we live in a high-tech world with access to a vast array of knowledge about how to stay healthy, and yet preventable noncommunicable diseases now account for more deaths worldwide than all other causes combined. We rarely hear about the person who dies peacefully in her sleep at ninety-nine years young. Instead, we hear about individuals who suffer mightily and eventually succumb after a long "battle."

In our age of information, where health tips are dispensed like candy by the media, the work of being healthy has gotten complicated. Just consider your own search for truth about what's good for you—or what's bad. It's common practice to rely on experts to tell us how to live—news stories covering the latest scientific findings, bestselling books that tout one theory or another, government recommendations, claims on labels, and doctors like me. But this advice is so terribly common that it commonly conflicts. What is a person to do with a hot media account of a new study that finds multivitamins effective in preventing cancer—only to read another media account the next day that says multivitamins can increase your risk for cancer and do nothing for heart health? (And to add insult to injury, you learn that the company that makes the vitamins is the same one that makes the drugs to combat cancer!)

When I wrote my first book, *The End of Illness*, my purpose was simple: to share what I'd learned from working out on the edge of the cliff that is the war on cancer—a place where we take risks in medicine in the hope of finding innovations to prolong people's lives. While the death rate from cancer hasn't changed dramatically in the past fifty years, progress against other diseases has relied on single discoveries that have allowed us to treat or eradicate them. Examples include the use of statins to prevent cardiovascular disease and stroke, antibiotics to combat infectious diseases originating from bacteria, antivirals and vaccines to tackle and protect against specific viruses, and a heightened awareness of the risks posed by behavioral factors such as smoking and poor diet or overeating. Except for these isolated improvements, why aren't we better at treating and curing chronic degenerative diseases that often cannot be blamed on a single culprit?

For decades we've tried to reduce our understanding of the body and its potential breakdowns to a finite cause, be it a mutation, a germ, a deficiency, or a number such as a white blood cell count, glucose level, or a triglyceride value. But this has led us far astray from a perspective that could not only change how we care for the body, but also how we create the next generation of treatments and, in some instances, cures. The original title of *The End of Illness*, upon which this life guide is based, was *What Is Health?* It's a question that bugs me and my colleagues to this day. I don't know what true health is. We can certainly try to measure health in a variety of ways—weight, cholesterol, blood sugar, blood cell count, how you look, and how well you sleep, for example. But that doesn't really tell me much in terms of overall health and how many years and days you might have left. This has motivated me to urge people to begin viewing their total health as a complex network of processes that cannot be explained by looking at any one pathway or focal point. In many instances, it does no good to try to understand a certain disease; we just need to control it, much like an air traffic controller manages planes without knowing exactly how to fly one. This radically different perspective on health is what can open the doorway to future solutions, and even cures.

I don't think I fully grasped the thorniness surrounding the subject of health, however, until I started discussing my book and responding to readers. I quickly found myself on the receiving end of questions like, What's your real motivation for writing a book? Why are you hawking prescription drugs? How can a doctor who treats the very rich have anything valuable to give the average person who barely has health insurance? Let me head this last question off at the pass right now by saying the vast majority of my "prescriptions" in this book are surprisingly simple, such as wearing good shoes (Rule 59) and eating lunch at the same time every day (Rule 3). How much does it cost to keep a fairly regular schedule every day and to walk around more (Rule 16)? Put another way, how much will you save by ditching your vitamins and supplements (Rule 62)? How much easier will your life get once you learn that it's better to buy frozen vegetables than some fresh produce (which isn't nearly as fresh as you think; see Rule 5). And even when I suggest something that comes with a price, such as paying for a DNA screening test, there's often an inexpensive, if not totally free, alternative (see Rule 19), which can be even more informative and useful.

When I went on the *Dr. Oz Show* in the fall of 2012, I was billed as the most controversial doctor in America. But I think I'm the absolute opposite. I won't endorse anything that's not backed by well-controlled clinical trials—studies that live up to the rigors of the scientific method. In that regard, I'm one of the most conservative of doctors in America. People tend to label certain things as aggressive or, conversely, mainstream. Many individuals think taking aspirin and statins on a daily basis is aggressive but taking vitamins is mainstream. But the data tell a totally different story, painting a picture in which aspirin and statins can significantly *reduce* your risk of death (what scientists call "all cause mortality") while vitamins and supplements may *raise* your risk for a variety of illnesses, including cancer. I can understand and appreciate someone's suspicion when hearing a doctor push a pill, and her assumption that there must be financial remuneration or incentive involved. For the record, I have no financial ties to any drug company. In the past I have been paid for giving lectures to pharmaceutical management teams, but I've never been involved with any pharmaceutical marketing. If I suggest a certain drug or class of drugs, it's for a good, well-documented reason: because they have been shown to make a positive difference.

I actually don't mind stirring up controversy and inspiring people to ask questions. Spending on food and health together make up more than 30 percent of the U.S. economy, yet our politicians and civic leaders aren't discussing these important issues. They may bicker about how to finance health-care reform, but I'd like to see more attention on the reform itself. It boggles my mind to think the conversation remains stuck on figuring out how to pay for health care rather than on diminishing our need for it. Indeed, part of my motivation in writing this book is to make you—the health-care consumer—an agent of change, starting with yourself. Each one of us can make a difference if we each are part of reducing the overall demand for health care. The result will follow one of the fundamental laws of Econ 101: when we start living strong, robust lives, we'll lessen our need for health care, causing the demand to decrease and costs to go down. Simple as that.

The other chief reason for writing this book is probably pretty obvious: I want these rules to reach as many people as possible. After *The End of Illness* came out, many people asked me to distill my Health Rules down to a prescriptive list for them to keep on hand. They wanted a cheat sheet. In my previous book, I spent a lot of time going through the evidence; I won't be doing that here. I also won't be using any medical terminology or fancy language to convey my ideas. This is as pure and direct as it gets—less about theory, research, history, and science and more about the basic practices you can follow in your daily life. Nothing is meant to be a rigid directive. Of all the rules I present, the most important one is this: you have to find what works for you. The sixty-five rules here are each accompanied by a paragraph or two of explanation. A few, however, require little or no clarification (Rule 29: Smile) and I hope you just accept them at face value.

My goal is that this book will allow you to take the confusion out of knowing how to live to be healthy—to feel as fabulous as possible at any age. As I said in my previous book:

My recommendations won't be terribly exacting. I'm not interested in telling you how to live your life or what you should be eating for dinner. I'm also not here to diagnose you. Instead, I want to empower you to take control over your body and the future of your health. The suggestions offered here are more like lifestyle algorithms—mental devices for thinking through our myriad lifestyle choices. Those choices must be tempered by our values and individual codes of ethics and behavior. Because there is no single answer to the question of what is health, these guidelines will produce as many different "healthy styles" as there are people living them.

My objective is to help you make the most of your health, whether or not you're currently battling an illness. I'd like to encourage you to take a hard look at your understanding of health and open up your mind to a change in perspective. It can significantly improve your life.

That we need simple reminders of what it means to live a healthy life despite the volume of advice transmitted daily in the media is a telling sign of our confusion. I can only hope that as you read this book you gain not only the knowledge you need to take advantage of modern science and medicine, but also the wisdom to discern the good from the questionable to make the best decisions for yourself. I also hope that your future will be determined by the power of choice, and, when necessary, that it will guide you down pathways of healing. Only you can end illness.

I've divided this book into three sections. The first, "What to Do," gives a clear set of just that—things you can do that will make you the architect of your health kingdom. The second part, "What to Avoid," offers my rules for the things to stay away from that can harm your health. Some of these will be obvious, such as limiting risky behaviors and avoiding less-than-perfect ingredients in foods, but some won't be so apparent, such as how not to fall prey to hyperbole in the media and how not to hoard your medical information. I'm going to help you learn how to separate the hype from the helpful and see the ways in which you can benefit from sharing your medical information with the world. Part three, "Doctor's Orders," makes my recommendations even more straightforward by listing out a plan based on which decade you're in (twenties, thirties, forties, and so on). This is your real cheat sheet—the bulleted list of agenda items you should tend to at each particular age. The nature of this book's structure and content makes for some repeated ideas, and two different rules may take you to the same place. My hope is that presenting these principles in different ways will make them more memorable. Enjoy the read, and I trust that a handful of these rules will stick with you and improve your life.

Before we begin, let me first present important ground rules.

Ground Rule 1

Health information is a moving target. Recommendations today may change tomorrow. For now, the following rules are relevant based on the data we have available that convincingly show the best practices for reducing your risk of disease. While it's true that you can find single, unrepeated studies that contradict my ideas, that's not how science works. When scientists weigh in on a topic, they can't just rely on single studies that support their view. Instead, they have to consider all the studies on a topic and examine the results of each. That is exactly what a meta-analysis does. Hence, all of my prescriptions are rooted in studies that meet this gold standard. They always will be. And if the day comes when science uproots an established "truth" or does a complete 180 on a universally accepted fact, then I will welcome that new viewpoint with excitement and resolve (and a new rule).

Ground Rule 2

The rules in this book are not meant to be blanket recommendations, especially when it comes to prescription medications. The point is to have a discussion about them with your doctor and family, and also to consider your inner core values. So take the time to sit, think, and talk through any new direction you decide to take in your life. Remember, too, that health is in constant flux (see Ground Rule 1). You need to adapt to changes as you age. In science-speak we say that humans are "emergent systems"—they are constantly changing, developing, and evolving. The body is an incredible self-regulating machine. You don't need to do much to support its health and optimal wellness. In the last hour, for instance, about one billion cells were replaced in your body without your having to think about it.

Ground Rule 3

You are in charge of you. This book is designed as a manual to help you know when to be introspective and when to question things. If I suggest something that offends you or that you flatly reject, just move on. At the heart of my message is the importance of knowing how to have a productive conversation with yourself and your physician; it's also about raising your awareness about the things you do today that affect your tomorrows. When you come across a rule that makes you feel uncomfortable, remember that none of these is absolutely perfect. Instead of dismissing it, ask for better studies and, in turn, better technology. We have to be pushing for progress. Here's a quick example: aspirin may be touted as a miracle drug (Rule 22), but it's still flawed, given the side effects it can cause, namely bleeding and upset stomach. We should question why the National Institutes of Health doesn't spend large sums on making better aspirin so we can reap its miraculous benefits minus the potential side effects.

One final confession: I admit that I was so moved by Michael Pollan's *Food Rules*, which was inspired by his bestselling *In Defense of Food: An Eater's Manifesto*, that his book provided the model for this one. I reference Pollan a few times in *The End of Illness*, for I deeply respect his take on dietary issues and think he states the facts brilliantly. So as much as *Food Rules* lays out a set of concise, memorable rules for eating wisely, my *Short Guide to a Long Life* similarly presents my set of rules for *living* wisely. This of course will include a few rules about eating and buying food, but I will also address all the other factors that play into good health. I've done my best to keep it short and sweet, while still keeping my promise to bestow on you the recipe for a long and healthy life.

PART I

—

What to Do

Listen, Look, Feel (and Record Your Body's Features)

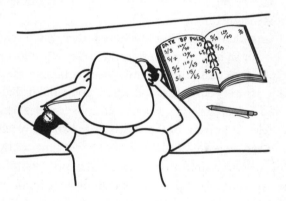

These days it's easier to know your blood pressure and heart rate than it is to find a pay phone. If I had to put one rule above all others, it would be this: get to know yourself. It's why I'm starting this entire list of things to do with a directive to take inventory of your body's features, characteristics, vital signs, and other health parameters that are relatively easy to obtain. Let's bring the concept of *listen, look, and feel*

home. Obviously, aim for the measurements you can take with tools at your fingertips or at a local pharmacy, or that don't require any hardware at all, just your inner thoughts and sensations. Include notes such as how you feel in general, how well you're sleeping, whether you harbor any aches and pains, and what kinds of activities or foods seem to irritate your body. How many of us never stop and ask: Do I feel healthy? Is it hard for me to get out of bed in the morning? Is there a pattern to the times when I feel lousy and, conversely, fantastic? You'd be surprised by how effortless it can be to decode the mysteries of your own body's quirks and rhythms just by tuning in!

If you want to get more technical, then gather clues to your body's signals by recording the following information daily over the course of three months: the time of day, your blood pressure, your pulse, and what's going on at that time (e.g., you just ate breakfast, you're anxious upon waking up, you're relaxed in front of the television, or you've received a piece of bad news in the mail). Pick different times of the day to do your self-examination, as this will inform you of times when, say, your blood pressure is high or your mood is low. You'll then want to repeat this exercise throughout the year, preferably once every couple of months, to note changes. Don't wait until you're in the doctor's office, which is typically a rare occasion for most of us. Do, however, bring your personal health diary with you to share at your next appointment. You can buy or access equipment to take your blood pressure at most pharmacies, and some tools can even be downloaded as an application for your smart phone (see Rule 2).

I'm a big believer in what's called personalized medicine, which means customizing your health care to your specific needs based on your physiology, genetics, value system, and individual circumstances. Medicine is finally at a place where we have the technology to tailor treatment and preventive protocols to an individual, just like a seamstress can tailor a garment to a person's body. But it all begins with you. You won't be able to enjoy the benefits of personalized medicine until you take a close look at your unique body.

Below is a list of general questions to ask yourself during your personal checkup every couple of months after you've completed the intense three-month initiation diary:*

- How would you rank your overall energy levels?
- Anything abnormal to report (skin, hair, sensations, breathing, appetite, digestion)?
- Do you suffer from any chronic conditions?
- How bad is your stress level on a scale of 1 to 10?
- Are you happy?
- What do you want to change in your life?
- What is your weight? (Aim to measure your weight once a week or every two weeks.)

Of course, these questions should also be asked on day 1. And be honest.

---

* Go to www.davidagus.com for a free comprehensive, downloadable questionnaire.

2 Measure Yourself

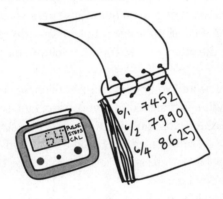

Every day I read about some new gadget or app on the market that can help track my health and happiness. (At last count, there were more than seven thousand self-tracking smart-phone apps alone, and the market for self-tracking gadgetry is exploding.)

How many steps did you take today? How long were you in dreamy REM sleep last night? How fast did you eat lunch? What's your pulse? How many calories are you burning? What's your blood oxygen level? What's your brain's electrical activity at night? How stressed are you? What emotions are you feeling? You can answer these questions if you have the right device. (Although I should hope you can take a good guess as to how stressed and emotional you are sans a digital reader.)

If you really want to take Rule 1 to the maximum, then consider measuring yourself a bit more formally with the help of nifty devices. In 2007, a couple of brainy *Wired* editors saw this coming: the day when we'd be able to track ourselves digitally as Sanctorius of Padua did manually when he weighed everything that came in and out of his body over a period of thirty years in the sixteenth and seventeenth centuries. The *Wired* editors coined the term the "quantified self," and this kind of effort has already become a movement. Even if you don't subscribe to the idea of wearing a piece of Star Treky equipment, most of us keep mental track of certain things in our lives such as weight, sleep quality, and activity level—if just to make sure we're within the parameters we'd like to follow.

But seriously, you might want to consider adding a tracking app or device of some kind to your life. I can't even begin to list them all here, and by the time you read this a whole new generation of useful software programs and devices will surely have hit the market. You can track, calculate, plan, and research just about anything health related these days and personalize that info. Some apps can be programmed for your location and, say, notify you of the foods in your geographical area that are in season and provide information on local farmers markets. Pretty soon we'll be able to wear little devices that can clue us in to our body's dynamics all day long. Not that we all may want to wear such gadgets 24/7, but these could be incredibly powerful tools for creating and maintaining baseline numbers, and in some cases for training ourselves to know when we could benefit from some behavioral modifications. It's hard to take yourself from a raging bull in terms of stress back down to a calm, cool cucumber, but if a device or app could alert you that you're entering a danger zone, it might motivate you to make effective changes to reduce your stress.

Tools are critical to our success in so many areas in life—e-mail and cell phones allow us to communicate, the Internet to research, cars to get where we are going. Why would we think that we don't need such help with our health? The tools are already at our disposal. They aren't meant to make us totally self-absorbed; they are meant to help us take better care of ourselves. Using them will propagate the incentives we need. Make it a goal to study yourself consistently and keep charts. Listen to your body, and remember—only you know your body best.

For a constantly updated list of interesting apps and devices, go to http://davidagus.com/mhealth.

3 Automate Your Life

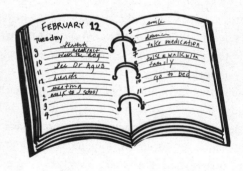

Your body loves predictability. Did you get up today at the same time as yesterday? Will you eat your next meal at roughly the same time you ate that meal yesterday? One of the best ways of reducing stress on your body and keeping its preferred, balanced state of being (homeostasis) is to maintain a regular, consistent routine on a daily basis, 365 days a year, to the best of your ability. Yes, regardless of weekends, holidays, social demands, late nights at the office, and other body-busting, schedule-disrupting events.

The four chief areas where you can make great strides in honoring your body's homeostasis are your sleep-wake cycles, eating times, periods of physical activity, and schedule for taking any prescribed medications. Just as your body aches for a consistent sleep schedule, it also craves a regular eating routine. If you were to step into a body that's been deprived of its expectation of eating lunch at noon, for example, you'd witness biological activities going on that would likely surprise you. Your body won't just show signs of hunger; it will also experience a surge in cortisol, the stress hormone that tells your body to hold tightly to fat and to conserve energy. In other words, if you don't eat when your body anticipates food, it will sabotage your efforts to lose or maintain an ideal weight.

By the same token, don't throw a wrench into that finely tuned body of yours by sporadic snacking or eating randomly when you're not hungry just to counteract an emotional state such as boredom, loneliness, or depression. If you don't normally snack at 3:00 p.m. every single day, then don't reach for that apple fritter to lift your late-afternoon lull. But if you need an afternoon snack, have it at a regular time. And go for a handful of nuts, a piece of whole fruit, veggies dipped in hummus, or some cheese and crackers rather than the processed fried dough.

4 Mobilize Your Medical Data

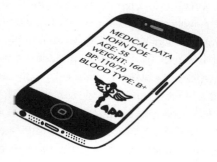

Do you have copies of all your medical records, and are they accessible online somewhere? Why not? What if you land in the emergency room and cannot talk but have a potentially fatal allergy to penicillin—the very drug a doctor is about to inject into you?

We use our phones and computers today for just about everything, with one exception: storing our medical records and keeping our health information updated. Aim to have all your records stored in your "mobile cloud" so they are always accessible to you. Give a trusted family member (spouse, parent, sibling, adult child) or friend your passwords so they can access those same files when and if it becomes necessary. Everyone needs a partner in health care. Pick someone. Give that person full access to all of the places where you keep your medical data. If you don't have your medical records nicely organized in digital files, request copies of your files from your doctors. Spend a weekend afternoon creating digital copies of them using a scanner. You can also keep them on a USB key chain that you take everywhere. This task may sound daunting, but it's just a few hours of work from which you can benefit for the rest of your life. It is unusual that patients of mine have a medical emergency between the hours of 9:00 a.m. and 5:00 p.m. when the office is open and we can access their records. Problems always seem to happen in the middle of the night, on a weekend, or when someone is traveling! We each have different health profiles, but that distinctiveness can present a challenge to doctors who don't know anything about us, yet have been given the job of treating us. Having your entire medical record on file to hand over just might save your life.

5 Eat Real Food (and Don't Let the Apple Fall Far from the Tree)

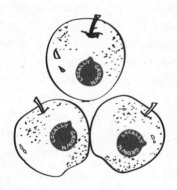

The best way to summarize the sad need for this rule is simply to quote Michael Pollan from his book *In Defense of Food*: "That anyone should need to write a book advising people to 'eat food' could be taken as a measure of our alienation and confusion."

And indeed, every day people ask the question, What should I eat?

Answer: real food.

What constitutes real food? With the exception of flash-frozen fruits and vegetables, anything that *doesn't* come with a label or an FDA-approved nutrition facts label is likely to be real, as ironic as that sounds. If you walk the perimeter of your grocery store (produce section, butcher, fishmonger), you'll find real food. Steer clear of those aisles lined with boxes and bottles and other food impostors that come in pretty packages. If you read a label that lists ingredients you cannot pronounce or define without a graduate-level textbook in chemistry, put that item back on the shelf and walk away! Focus on consuming foods that are as close to nature as possible, which will also help you to avoid problematic ingredients that you don't know you're sensitive to.

Watch out for health claims, too. If a food product has to tell you that it's good for you (with descriptions and health claims on their packaging that say things like "low fat!" "low in sugar!" "lite," "cholesterol free!" "baked not fried," "antioxidant rich," and "all natural"), then it's probably not very real. Think about it: in order for claims to be made, the food must be packaged somehow and pass some sort of test or criteria for the seal of approval. This means that the food cannot possibly be all that real and as close to nature as possible. Orange juice, for instance, will come with lots of health claims ("a full day's worth of vitamin C!"), but the quiet, lonely whole orange sitting in a produce basket will do more for your health than an eight-ounce glass of fiberless fructose. If they have to tell you why you should be eating it, you *shouldn't* be eating it. What's more, many people think they are eating healthily when they buy diet frozen dinners, fat-free ice cream or frozen yogurt, 100 percent natural fruit juice, low-fat cheese, energy bars, diet soda, organic hundred-calorie snack packs, and so on. But if you look at the nutritional content of these foods, and the order in which the ingredients are listed, which reflects their prevalence, you're likely to find more sugar, saturated fat, salt, and ingredients with weird names than anything else.

And one more note about this rule: go for seasonal items when you buy fresh produce. If you find yourself eating blueberries and heirloom tomatoes in February or brussels sprouts and kiwifruit in June, then you're likely eating fruits and veggies that have fallen too far from the tree. In other words, they have traveled a long way to get to your GPS coordinates. The minute a fruit or vegetable is picked is the moment it starts to change chemically and lose nutritional value. Too many fruits and vegetables are available year-round now thanks to shipping technologies. We may live in a world where we can access pretty much any type of food all year long, but it comes at a major expense: nutrition. By the time the vast majority of produce reaches the bins and aisles of your local supermarket, it doesn't contain nearly the same amount of nutrients as when plucked from the plant or yanked from its roots. If fruits and vegetables are picked before they are ripe—which many of them are to help them endure the long shipment—they have less time to develop a full spectrum of vitamins and minerals. The produce might look ripe on the outside, but it will never have the same nutritive value as it would have if it had been allowed to ripen fully before harvest. In addition, during the long haul from farm to fork, fresh fruits and vegetables are exposed to lots of heat and light, which also degrade some nutrients, especially delicate vitamins such as C and the B vitamin thiamine. What we end up with in our mouths is a nutrient-poor product that may also contain some chemicals that we would like to avoid.

Unless you can buy truly fresh produce that's in season and has been delivered recently from a nearby farm, head on over to your grocer's freezer section and opt for frozen fruits and vegetables, often labeled as "fresh flash-frozen." Fruits and vegetables chosen for freezing tend to be plucked or picked at their peak ripeness, a time when—as a general rule—they are packed with the most nutrients. Eat fruits and vegetables soon after purchase, including the frozen variety. Over many months, even the nutrients in frozen vegetables inevitably degrade. And for produce that you can buy truly fresh, please don't insult the sweet fruit and vibrant veggies by letting them languish in your kitchen's fruit bowl or crisper in the refrigerator. Enjoy them as soon as possible.

All of this leads us to the question, How can you know what's truly fresh? Ah, see the next rule.

6 Know Your Grocer

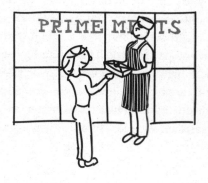

Short of being a farmer who knows exactly what's in season, you can learn all the information you need to make smart purchases just by chatting up your local grocer. The people who stock the produce section, for instance, will tell you what just came in, where it came from, and how it was farmed. The guy manning the butcher counter can share details about the ranchers who supplied the meat, and the woman behind the fish counter can offer information as to which fish is the freshest, most sustainably caught. Don't be intimidated by these folks. They love imparting their knowledge.

And when you do venture out of the grocery store and into your local farmers market, that's where you'll want to introduce yourself to the people who are that much closer to the source of your food. Get to know your local farmers as you would your grocer. Farmers markets rarely sell imported items, so what you find there will be the freshest possible. If you can buy most of your fresh produce from a local farmers market, you can automatically avoid the nutrient-poor, processed, nonseasonal fare. You may have to spend a little more for your groceries, but this is when it really counts. You get what you pay for: you'll be eating high-quality foods and enjoying a high quality of life that won't cost you bundles in health-care bills for illnesses you could have avoided. Besides, high-quality food just tastes better, so you're more likely to be satisfied with less of it, thereby controlling your calories.

7 Grow a Garden

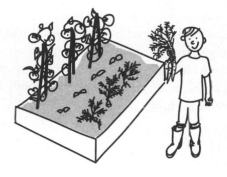

This should be a mandatory rule for anyone with children, especially young ones. I know of no better way to teach principles of health and good eating than to show kids what real food looks like in the growing phase. This will force you to learn what blooms in May versus what crops up in December. And there's just nothing you can buy in the grocery store or even at your farmers market that compares nutritionwise with food you pick a few feet from your kitchen and use immediately for cooking or just eat raw.

Don't panic if you live in an itty-bitty apartment or lack a green thumb. Be willing to experiment and start with easy plants that work in your climate and space. Your local nursery will be able to give you all the details and equipment you need (think pots, soil, seeds). You needn't own an acre or have a huge amount of unused area in your yard. A simple window box will suffice. And you can just start by growing herbs and spices (parsley, basil, mint, sage), then graduate to some of the more advanced crops as your space allows, such as peppers, tomatoes, cucumbers, green beans, snow peas, lettuce, and Swiss chard. In some places, you can grow a garden all year round and rotate which crops you're cultivating based on the season. Better yet, make this a community effort and join forces with neighbors. Split up who grows what and share in the bounty. Now, that's neighborly for a good cause: community health.

8 Maintain a Dietary Protocol That Works for You

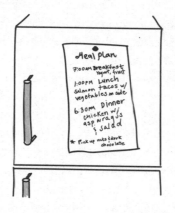

Should you eat gluten free? Low carb? Vegan? Raw? Low fat? Follow Weight Watchers? In truth, it doesn't really matter as long as you enjoy what you're eating, your body seems to love it, and you're not forcing yourself to adhere to an impossibly strict protocol that probably lacks certain nutrients by virtue of its restrictions. Just as there are many religions in the world, there are many healthy eating traditions, and it is worth remembering why they have worked through the centuries.

I love how Michael Pollan puts it in his forty-eighth food rule: "Eat More Like the French. Or the Japanese. Or the Italians. Or the Greeks." Any traditional diet will beat out our processed food culture, and traditional eating habits have worked for centuries among different peoples (with vastly different diets) around the world. These habits include moderating portions, sharing food at a communal table, not going back for seconds, and letting hunger build up in between meals (no snacking). Today, a great part of our larger-than-life waistlines is due not only to poor dietary choices but also to poor eating habits. We eat in solitude on the go, in our cars, and at our desks. Seldom do we sit around the table and linger over lively conversations with loved ones. And we go back for second and third (and fourth) helpings as if the food is unlimited (because it pretty much is). We also avoid the sensation of hunger by eating randomly throughout the day, mindlessly downing lots of snacks. Or, on the other end of the spectrum, if we skip meals and save our caloric load for a banquet at night, we're more likely to overindulge and then have trouble sleeping. So always leave the dinner table a little hungry (and leave something on your plate—a clean plate is not always a happy plate!).

One of the easiest ways to gain control of the ideal diet for you is simply to cook more. Make your own food. Enjoy it with others at a table (not a desk, in front of the television, or behind the wheel). Borrow recipes from around the world and buy fresh ingredients. I'll even give you permission to eat as many snack foods and delectable desserts as you like so long as you make them from scratch using real ingredients and have them at a daily regular snack time. Then abide by the same portion control rules you'd use for any regular meal, treating treats as treats, and you'll have accomplished more than the vast majority of Americans.

9 Cultivate Om in the Office

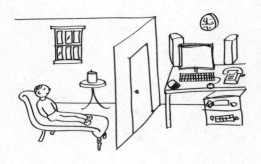

It shouldn't take a study to highlight the negative impact work-related stress can have on us physically, but now we can point to several, one of which was done recently in Finland that showed just how bad job stress can be. In 2012, Finnish researchers examined nearly three thousand people and correlated stress on the job with faster biological aging. How exactly did they calculate this? They measured these people's telomeres—DNA sequences found at the end of a person's chromosomes and whose lengths can be associated with aging, risk of illness, and possibly death. The theory put simply is that the shorter your telomeres, the shorter your life. And it turns out that the more pressure you feel at work, the more likely that your telomeres will shorten. In addition to this correlative relationship on your telomeres, there is the increased risk for heart trouble when you carry so much stress. It's practically cliché now to say that stress causes heart disease, but it's true. The heart may be among the strongest, most invincible organs in our body—after all, it pumps about 2,000 gallons of blood each day and beats, on average, more than 100,000 times daily—but that doesn't mean it's immune to things as subtle as psychological stress. It's no surprise that we're most likely to suffer a heart attack on a Monday, the first day of the workweek.

Job strain is a part of life. So what can we do to ease the pressure? Maintain simple routines at work that lift your mood and keep things in perspective. Some ideas: go for a walk during lunch in the bright sun; walk around more in the office and take your calls while standing up and moving around; take a deep breath before answering the phone; play relaxing music while working; skip happy hour and go to the gym to burn off steam instead; take scheduled time-outs during the day when you visit your favorite blogger or web-site for a few minutes; and decide when you check e-mail and respond to messages. The average working professional spends roughly 23 percent of the workday on e-mail and glances at the inbox about thirty-six times an hour. It takes most of us more than a minute to return to a task once we've stopped to read a new e-mail. And that can add stress.

10 Have a Glass of Wine with Dinner

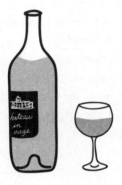

Habits that transcend culture and religion and date back thousands of years probably have some benefit to them regardless of what the science says. But now we know that moderate alcohol intake, especially from red wine, can reduce one's risk for heart disease. This benefit does have a caveat, however: drinking can potentially increase one's risk for breast cancer, and drinking too much is far worse for your heart than being a teetotaler. How do you find the sweet spot? Aim for no more than one drink a day if you're a woman and two if you're a man. And if you abstain during the workweek, you don't have permission to binge drink over the weekend.

11 Practice Good Hygiene— in Bed and Out

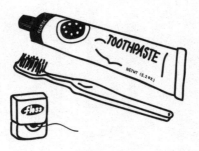

Good health starts with good hygiene. It's hard to believe that the dramatic decrease in infectious diseases between the discovery of germs and antidotes such as antibiotics and vaccines was actually not the result of high-tech medical treatments, but rather of changes in how we practice good hygiene. Although technically not a discovery on par with penicillin and the smallpox or polio vaccines, the mid-nineteenth-century recognition of the importance of hand washing was a huge medical breakthrough that saved a lot of people long before vaccines and antibiotics were widely available.

In 1847, while working at an obstetrics clinic in Vienna, Hungarian-born physician Dr. Ignaz Semmelweis noticed that fatal fevers among mothers of newborn children happened more frequently in birthings assisted by medical students than in those assisted by midwives. This prompted him to look closer at the clinic's practices, and he soon noted that the medical students who aided in childbirth often did so after performing autopsies on people who had died from bacterial sepsis—a whole-body blood infection in which the inflammatory response to a blooming bacteria turns deadly. He then established a strict policy of hand washing with a chlorinated antiseptic solution, and lo and behold, mortality rates dropped ten- to twentyfold within three months. It was proof that the transfer of disease could be significantly reduced by this simple hygienic practice, even though doctors at the time didn't know the exact causes of such diseases in many cases. Had civilization figured this out sooner, perhaps we could have avoided many of the deaths associated with plagues and epidemics that wiped out millions of people in earlier centuries.

Even today, we are inclined to trivialize the simple act of hand washing and would do well to keep it at the top of our priorities on a daily basis. You'll give yourself an advantage in avoiding germs that can make you sick, and you'll help prevent the spread of germs to others. All you need is a dollop of soap and water. Antimicrobial soaps aren't necessary; the standard stuff is just as good. But if you don't have access to water, then use an alcohol-based hand sanitizer. Some studies have shown that people who washed their hands at least five times a day were 35 percent less likely to catch the flu than those who lathered up less.

In addition to hand hygiene, maintaining general hygiene throughout your body will go a long way to protect you from the ick factor—think about head lice, bad breath, body odor, pinworms, and athlete's foot. All of these can largely be controlled just by practicing good hygiene. Don't forget to tend to cuts and scrapes immediately with antiseptics and bandages, no matter how trivial they seem. This will help you to avoid dangerous skin infections such as a painful staph invasion from hard-to-kill bacteria that can require serious oral antibiotics later on. And what about bed hygiene? Restful sleep starts with a clean and tidy bedroom. Wash your sheets in hot water once a week and keep clutter and electronics out. This habit will help you to practice good sleep hygiene (see Rule 58).

12 Cohabitate

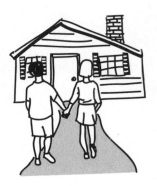

While at first blush it may seem unlikely that a connection has been found between cohabitation and longevity, consider the following: when you live with someone else, you have a reason to pay more attention to your health and hygiene. You've got another person to hold you accountable for your actions and lifestyle habits. You're less likely to engage in risky behaviors. And you're more likely to have a built-in system for coping with stress, because another warm human body is present in your daily life. If you come home mad, frustrated, and on the verge of a breakdown, you've at least got a sounding board. Which might explain why happy co-habitating couples repeatedly score better on blood pressure tests than their single counterparts. Whether or not this rule should entail marriage is up to you. And whether it should include children is another thing to consider (see Rule 47).

13 Maintain a Healthy Weight

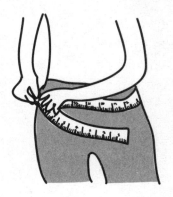

It should come as no surprise that a healthy weight corresponds to a healthy body. When the body is saddled with too many pounds (or, on the other end of the spectrum, too few pounds), it cannot function optimally. Here's another way to look at it: each pound of weight lost equals a four-pound reduction in the knee load for every step you take. So if you take ten thousand steps a day, that translates to a twenty-ton reduction in the pressure on your knees. Think of that cumulative effect over a whole year! Even a small weight loss makes a big difference in the long run.

Being overweight increases your risk for virtually all illnesses and chronic conditions, from the obvious ones like heart disease, arthritis, and diabetes to dementia and cancer. Don't know if you're at a healthy weight? Search for a body mass index (BMI) calculator and chart online and see how you match up. The goal is to maintain a BMI of between 18.5 and 24.9. The National Heart, Lung and Blood Institute has a good one at http://nhlbisupport.com/bmi.

14 Get Your Annual Flu Shot, Even If You "Never Get Sick" and "Have Never Gotten the Flu"

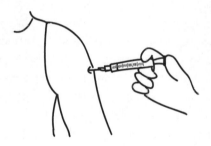

If you could take an inexpensive pill once a year that would help prevent all forms of cancer and has zero side effects, you'd probably consider it. Well, that's what a flu shot has the potential to do. It's a simple annual vaccine that will go a long way in protecting you from getting terribly sick for days, if not weeks, during which you cannot work, focus, fulfill your household duties, hang out with family members and friends, and enjoy life as usual. But immunizing yourself against influenza isn't just about beating the flu. A mere one to two weeks of an inflammatory storm, which is what will take place in your body if you contract the flu, can harm you in ways that increase your lifetime risk for obesity and many illnesses, including heart attack, strokes, and cancer.

For years now the American Heart Association and the American College of Cardiology have recommended flu vaccines for anyone with heart disease because it's been shown to prevent fatal heart attacks and strokes and even reduce the risk of death from any illness. In 2012, a study emerged showing that pregnant women who suffer through the flu have a significantly increased risk of having a child with autism. So imagine what the vaccine can do for a healthy individual hoping to avoid all these ills. (An idea: since we know the flu shot can lessen the risk for obesity, perhaps we should campaign for it by saying it will keep you thin! How many people would show up at the immunization clinic?) Sadly, people still cling to false notions that the flu vaccine has side effects, that it doesn't work, that it can *cause* the flu, or that it contains toxins or poisons. Malarkey. Most disturbing of all is that the people who seem to harbor these irrational notions are often the most educated. To say "I never get a flu shot and I never get the flu" is like declaring "I eat cheeseburgers and fries every day, don't exercise, and I've never gotten fat or had a heart attack."

There is nothing heroic about resisting the flu shot and then powering through the flu if you contract it. Influenza kills as many as forty-five thousand Americans a year, and the vaccine reduces deaths, illnesses, the use of antibiotics, and the number of hospital visits. Getting the shot isn't just about you; it can greatly lessen the burdens on our health-care system and can protect the most vulnerable of all—infants, the elderly, and people with weakened immune systems—who cannot benefit from the shot the way most of us can. To hear that fewer than 40 percent of us get an annual flu shot is maddening. Who wants to be blamed for fueling an epidemic and killing young children? I rest my case.

15 Get Naked

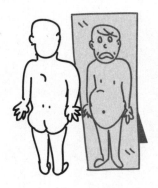

We throw our clothes on and off daily, during which time we're partially or wholly naked for a few seconds or minutes, and we spend quality time in the shower in our birthday suit. But when was the last time you took a good look at yourself butt naked in front of a mirror—front and back? You'd be surprised by how illuminating this exercise can be. You can spot trouble on the horizon in the form of body oddities that you didn't have before and signs of skin cancer. The skin acts as an indicator of the state of the entire body, and external skin discolorations, blemishes, lesions, rashes, blotches, or other unsightly marks can be signs of underlying internal disease. Once in a while, take a visual inventory of every square inch of yourself, including your hair, nails, and the inside of your mouth.

You can also get an honest sense of how well you are aging based on your physical appearance alone. Is your overall skin tone and set of wrinkles reflective of someone your age? Do you look older than your chronological age? And you can use this moment to gather measurements that can help you track the progress you're making by changing your habits. Measure your waist and see it get smaller. Start a skin-care routine that nourishes the health of your skin (and keeps you examining your skin regularly). Or maybe just tell yourself that you're beautiful and doing okay. Say an affirmation as you stand there naked and accept who you are. We all know that having a strong sense of self and being comfortable in our own skin will go a long way to keeping us healthy and psychologically strong.

16 Get Off Your Butt More

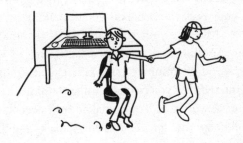

If you're a construction worker, farmer, baggage handler at the airport, or someone whose job is physically intense (in other words, you spend much of the day upright exerting yourself physically), you get a free pass on this rule and can move on to the next. But if you're like most people, you spend a great deal of time sitting as a result of your desk job, long commute, penchant for the couch, or the mere fact that you're getting older and sitting more seems inevitable. There's no end to the number of studies that prove the power of exercise in maintaining health, including a profound link between more time spent sitting and greater incidence of obesity, diabetes, cardiovascular disease, and even greater total mortality. One of the first studies ever done that pointed to the value of regular physical activity—"regular" meaning throughout the day—came out of a comparison of London's double-decker bus drivers and ticket takers in the 1950s. The ticket takers, who climbed up and down stairs all day as part of their job, had a much lower incidence of heart attacks than the bus drivers, who sat most of the day. Provocative recent studies show that physical activity even has antiaging effects on our DNA. It's true that you can change the expression of your genes—tipping the scales in favor of a long, robust life—just by getting off your bottom more. Is it any wonder that in the last century, as desk jobs became more prevalent, we witnessed a concomitant rise in illnesses related to being sedentary?

By the way, sitting itself is not the culprit here; it's the biological effects that sitting triggers in the body. Just as exercise spurs positive metabolic changes to our body, being inactive causes metabolic changes in the opposite, negative direction. And prolonged time spent sitting, *independent of how much other physical activity is done during the day,* has been shown to have significant metabolic consequences, negatively influencing such things as blood fats, cholesterol, blood sugar, resting blood pressure, and the appetite hormone leptin, all of which are risk factors for obesity, cardiovascular illness, and other chronic diseases.

Something else to keep in mind: if you think that you're doing your body good when you fit in an hour-long workout before or after a long day at your desk, think again. Even two hours of exercise a day will not compensate for spending twenty-two hours sitting on your derriere or lying in bed. No matter how much you sweat it out during a daily hard-core workout (or, God forbid, save it all for the weekend), if you're routinely sitting for hours at a time, you may as well be smoking. That's more or less the impact that prolonged sitting will have on your health risks. So get up and get moving—more! It's the only proven fountain of youth.

17 Jack Your Heart Rate Up 50 Percent Above Your Resting Baseline for at Least Fifteen Minutes Every Day

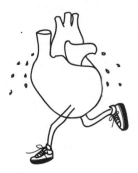

To reap the benefits of exercise, including all those biochemical reactions that take place to lower your risk of illness and keep your body humming, aim for breaking a sweat and getting your heart pumping fast for a minimum of fifteen minutes a day. We know now that the old guidelines recommending about a half hour of exercise five days a week are just that—old. If you stick with that minimum, you won't stop weight gain as you get older unless you really scale back the caloric intake. And even if you do achieve weight management through diet alone, that's beside the point. Unless you move your body and force your lungs and heart to work harder, you don't experience all the health-boosting pluses that exercise offers, from reducing your risk of heart disease to minimizing the chances that you'll become obese, diabetic, and depressed. In the long run, routinely breaking a sweat will do more for your happiness than routinely eating slices of chocolate cake (and not exercising).

And if you needed one more reason to push yourself physically, consider this: a high-intensity workout could make you smarter. On average, there are 100 billion neurons in each of our brains, and they love a good physical workout. Studies now show that older people who still do vigorous exercise, play competitive sports, or just walk several times a week protect their brains' white matter from shrinking. So if you plan to have a superbly functioning brain in your golden years, and dodge the evils of senility and Alzheimer's disease, then commit to an exercise routine. It can be as simple as leisurely walking.

18 Start a Sensible Caffeine Habit

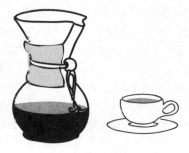

As with moderate drinking, consuming caffeine in moderation from natural sources like the coffee bean and tea leaf has long been shown to confer positive benefits on our health. Anecdotal evidence alone tells us that caffeine helps us feel energetic, alert, and upbeat. It can even help us to run faster or cycle quicker, which is why coffee is often the beverage of choice for runners and cyclists before races. This is due to caffeine's stimulating effects on the cardiovascular and central nervous systems. It prepares the brain and body for action by triggering an increase in heart rate, dilating your body's 60,000 miles of blood vessels to ease blood flow, and boosting sensitivity to stimulation. Although researchers have tried to link caffeine consumption with illnesses such as heart disease, hypertension, osteoporosis, and cancer, study after study has proven otherwise. Caffeine, especially from traditional sources and not modern, factory-made concoctions that sell as energy drinks, may actually have protective anticancer properties. But, again, moderation is key.

Too much of a good thing will turn ugly, as overconsuming caffeine can make you prone to anxiety, headaches, migraines, feeling jittery, and more. And while rare, caffeine overdosing can happen if you imbibe some of today's concentrated energy drinks. Slowly sipping a hot coffee is not the same as quickly downing a shot that's loaded with caffeine and probably sugar, too. So enjoy your coffee or tea and avoid the more processed jolts. Cut back on caffeine in the afternoon, especially after 2:00 p.m. Your body needs time to process all the caffeine so it won't infringe upon restful sleep. If you need a pick-me-up late in the day, then at least opt for tea since it has less caffeine. Or go for a walk.

19 Ask Mom or Dad What Killed Grandpa and Aunt Marge

FAMILY HISTORY

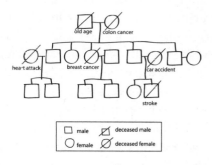

Did your grandparents die of "old age"? The last time you had to fill out a health history questionnaire in the doctor's office and you encountered questions about relatives and whether or not *anyone* in your family suffered from heart disease, dementia, or cancer, did you find yourself scratching your head? Asking our parents and other family members about the diseases in our bloodline is not an easy thing to do. But it can be more effective at helping us prevent illness than any technical test performed by a lab. In fact, family history is one of the most underused but powerful tools for understanding your health. And it's the surest way to escape more invasive tests. So buck up and ask the tough questions. All it costs is a little time questioning your relatives. Fewer than a third of families maintain a good, updated health tree, yet the Cleveland Clinic has proven that learning about your family tree is one of the best genetic tools to predict cancer risks.

If querying mom or dad and your favorite uncle over the phone sounds daunting, then make it a goal to initiate the conversation at your next family gathering. Reunions, holidays, and even funerals can make for ideal times to talk. The U.S. surgeon general operates a free website—https://familyhistory.hhs.gov—that will help you to create a family health history and share it electronically with relatives and your doctor. One word of caution: be sure to obtain information from both sides of the family, especially if you're a woman who knows less about your paternal relatives than those from your mother's side. A higher risk for breast or ovarian cancer can originate from either side of the family.

20 Consider DNA Testing

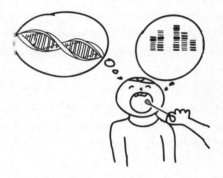

So your grandfather died of a heart attack in his fifties and your mom was diagnosed with colon cancer in her forties. What should you take from that bit of information? You might want to have your heart and colon checked out using the latest technology when you celebrate your fortieth birthday, if not sooner. The government maintains recommendations of when we all should get screened for this and that, but a much better way to know when and if you should ask for certain tests is to have an idea of your individual risks from family history. And if you wish for as much accuracy as possible, you can further add to that library of knowledge by spitting into a tube and getting your DNA screened.

Currently, we can look at genetic risk profiles for about forty conditions, from aneurysms to multiple sclerosis to stomach cancer. A small handful of companies have emerged that conduct genetic testing. I'm a firm believer in the power of this technology, which will continue to have more utility as we add more medical conditions to the existing list and learn about new associations between DNA variants and certain illnesses. The test won't only tell you what your DNA says about your risks; it can also clue you in to how your body metabolizes drugs and substances like caffeine and alcohol.

These tests do cost several hundred dollars, but once you pay for them, you'll gain access through the Internet to ongoing information relevant to you and based on new research. (Many of the companies that conduct the testing allow you to have an online account where you can keep track of new science that pertains to your unique DNA.) You'll also learn how you can modify your current behavior to reduce your risk of conditions you may be susceptible to and identify what's important to tell your doctor. In some cases, your genetic code can indicate whether you are likely to experience severe side effects from a particular drug, or whether the drug is likely to be effective, or how to dose the drug perfectly for you. By knowing how you are likely to respond to certain medications, you and your doctor can work together to make the right choices.

One of the more powerful tools that DNA screening provides is sheer motivation. I can tell you that you have a 30 percent chance of becoming obese based on the rate of obesity in the general population, which is probably white noise to you. But if your DNA could inform you that your risk of becoming obese in your lifetime is 60 to 80 percent, based on your genetics, this would likely mean something, wouldn't it? That might be enough to inspire you to pay more attention to the habits that affect your weight. Another way to look at it: if you knew that your personal risk for having a fatal heart attack in your life was 90 percent, you'd probably do everything you could to treat your heart well.

The combination of your DNA profile and the history you glean from family members can ultimately answer a lot of questions for you: Should you have a glass of wine with dinner? Should you get a mammogram before you turn forty? Can you wait until you're fifty to undergo your first colonoscopy? Is a stress test on your heart a good idea now? When should you consider taking a statin and baby aspirin? Should you be on the lookout for diabetes? Is a switch from participating in multiple marathons a year to a few half marathons a good idea given your age and risk for joint problems?

Because there is no one size fits all in medicine, it pays to be able to answer questions like these.

21 Inquire About Statins If You're Over the Hill

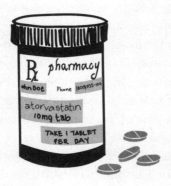

Heart disease still remains the number one killer of Americans, trailed closely by cancer and then stroke. Age-adjusted death rates from cardiovascular disease have declined 60 to 70 percent since 1950 thanks to advances in technology (including the use of statins) and better education about diet, exercise, and the risks of smoking. But the vast majority of us are still going to die of heart disease, stroke, or cancer either at a ripe old age or sooner if we don't take preventive measures. For a long time we thought statins were targeting only cholesterol, and that by reducing the body's production of cholesterol they were responsible for lowering one's risk for heart disease. But it turns out that they have a profound effect on the entire body. Statins have the power to change the whole environment by lowering inflammation—a biological process that can run amok and trigger all kinds of dysfunctions and illnesses.

To be clear, statins are compounds that inhibit a liver enzyme that plays a central role in the production of cholesterol. They are among the most commonly prescribed drugs in medicine to improve blood cholesterol levels in people who cannot control their cholesterol through diet alone, and they include such brands as Lipitor and Crestor. Statin compounds can be derived synthetically or isolated from naturally occurring foods such as red yeast rice and oyster mushrooms. But as I've already mentioned, statins don't just affect cholesterol.

When a body has high levels of inflammation markers, it means that it's encountering harmful stimuli, which can be any number of things from germs to damaged cells to irritants. To protect itself, the body triggers inflammation, an elaborate response involving the vascular system, the immune system, and various cells within the injured tissue. Researchers are now discovering bridges between certain kinds of inflammation and our most pernicious degenerative diseases, including Alzheimer's disease, cancer, autoimmune diseases, diabetes, and an accelerated aging process in general. Virtually all chronic conditions have been linked to chronic inflammation.

The first study to point out the value of statins in reducing inflammation came out of Harvard in 2008. It showed that taking these drugs could dramatically lower the risk of first-time heart attacks, strokes, and other artery problems in healthy men over fifty and women over sixty years of age who do not have high cholesterol but have high levels of inflammation markers—a sign that something isn't right and that the body is experiencing lots of widespread inflammation.

We know now that the real underlying reason for cardiovascular events may not be all about cholesterol, and that chronic inflammation is likely the cause. We also know that statins may not be all about preventing heart trouble. Since 2008, numerous other studies from impressively large controlled populations have demonstrated that statins can significantly lower our risk from dying of *anything*—cancer included. (Case in point: the *New England Journal of Medicine* published a study in 2012 involving 300,000 people that chronicled a dramatically lowered risk of death from cancer among those who took statins.)

Is a statin for everyone? Probably not. But it's worth a discussion with your doctor if you're over forty years old. In fact, pose the question as follows: "Doc, why *shouldn't* I be on a statin?"

22 Take a Baby Aspirin

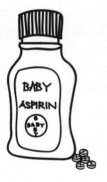

It's one of the oldest remedies known to mankind. Hippocrates, the father of modern medicine, used aspirin's active ingredient, salicylic acid, which he extracted from the bark and leaves of the willow tree, to help alleviate pain and fevers. In 1897, the German chemist Felix Hoffmann developed the first commercially available aspirin for Bayer, and since then, this wonder drug has proved its value as an effective, trusty analgesic.

Today we know that aspirin has far-reaching effects on the body as a whole that go beyond easing our headaches and sore backs. Many high-quality research studies have confirmed that the use of aspirin not only substantially reduces the risk of cardiovascular disease, but it can even ward off a medley of ailments through its anti-inflammatory powers. A daily low-dose aspirin (75 milligrams; similar to the more commonly available dose in the United States of 81 milligrams) has even been shown to reduce the risk of developing common malignant cancers in the lungs, colon, and prostate by a staggering 46 percent. So if you're basking in the glory of middle age, this might be something you'll want to discuss with your doctor (as there are side effects to aspirin such as bleeding that are real). It's the cheapest fountain of youth around and requires no prescription.

23 Abide by Screening and Booster Vaccination Recommendations

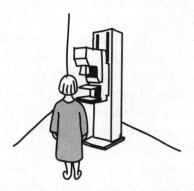

When our children are born, we take them to the pediatrician like clockwork for their regular checkups, and we (and the government) insist on vaccinating them for the measles, mumps, rubella, and polio. Why? Because we know these preventive strategies save lives. But as adults, we tend to get lazy and cavalier about keeping up with our own screenings and receiving booster shots. But this allows you to take advantage of the power of preventive medicine.

If you consider the major cancer killers in men, the top three are prostate, lung, and colon cancer. Together they represent almost 60 percent of deaths from cancer. If you're a man, prostate specific antigen (PSA) tests can identify prostate cancer early through a simple blood sample. If the subsequent prostate biopsy reveals that you have a form of high-risk prostate cancer, then you may benefit from treatment, whether that means surgery or radiation therapy. In the case of lung cancer, giving up cigarettes and minimizing your exposure to secondhand smoke can certainly decrease your risk for this type of cancer, and chest CT screenings can further decrease your chance of death from this disease. Colon cancer can similarly be avoided through colonoscopies that identify and remove polyps prior to their becoming cancerous. If you're a woman, the top cancer killers are those of the breast, lung, and colon. Again, you can help prevent and treat all of these with current screening tools, which have a profound impact on your chances of ever dying from these diseases.

Whether you're a man or a woman, preventing or delaying heart disease and stroke is also relatively straightforward and doable. We now know how certain dietary rules and the use of statins and baby aspirin, where appropriate, can come into play. You can also undergo a stress test for your heart, among other readily available tests, if you're at high risk for heart disease.

And don't forget about your booster shots and adult

vaccines. Science has developed a panoply of new vaccines that weren't available to our parents, and they can help us to avoid things like whooping cough, shingles, certain kinds of pneumonia, and hepatitis B. Of course, your age and risk factors will determine when and if you need them. But ask! And if you're a parent of a teenager, inquire about the vaccine against the human papillomavirus (HPV). Immunizing your adolescent against this ubiquitous virus will help dramatically reduce his or her lifetime risk of various cancers.

24 Plan a One-, Five-, Ten-, and Twenty-Year Health Strategy

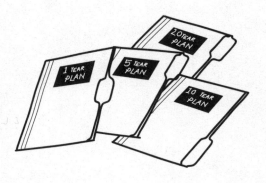

We all need goals. They help us to stay focused and give us something to look forward to. It's common to create goals for our professional pursuits and personal dreams such as buying a home and starting a family. But what about those other goals that have everything to do with our longevity and, let's face it, our ability to achieve *any* goal. Granted, lots of people resolve to lose weight every year, but that goal eludes most people. It's hard to lose weight when the weight goal is specific but the plan is not. Better to design a one-, five-, ten-, and twenty-year health strategy. Where do you see yourself in twenty years from a health perspective? What will you look like if you keep on the same path you're on now? What do you *want* to look like? It's hard to picture ourselves that far in the future, but it can help inform the choices we make today. So devise a plan and then work backward. Come up with little milestones you can achieve on that path. Instead of saying, "I will lose weight," reframe that goal to include the measures you'll take to get there. For example, "I will work out at least five days a week for thirty minutes at a time"; "I will remove 80 percent of processed foods from my diet"; "I will see my doctor once a year for a routine checkup."

As you think about where you want to be in a year, and then in five, ten, and twenty years, consider more than just your physical looks (although that's often a telltale sign of overall health and wellness). Reflect on your entire family while you're at it. Will you be able to keep up with your kids (and possibly grandkids) two decades from now? What steps can you take to ensure that you're able to take care of your spouse, who already has a chronic condition today? In five years, which risk factors will you need to pay extra attention to, given your age then? And in ten years, if you could look back to today, what would you want to do differently?

25 Deal with Sickness Smartly

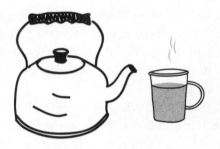

We all do it: cuddle up in bed with the shades drawn when we're nursing a bad cold or stomach virus. But part of the art of dealing with sickness means sticking to our routines as much as possible. Lying in bed all day in the dark might not be what's best for us if we want a quick recovery. Our lymph system, after all, plays a big part in fighting infections, but it won't send out its germ-fighting troops unless the body is mobile. So walk around when you're under the weather. Keep your body's internal clock on time by exposing it to the daylight; avoid creating a nighttime setting when the sun is out or you'll throw your body's circadian rhythm out of whack and give it another challenge to overcome in addition to illness.

When you feel a cold coming on (say, the beginnings of a scratchy throat), start sucking on zinc lozenges (more specifically, zinc acetate, the form of the metal most effective at fighting colds). Zinc—not echinacea or vitamin C—is about the only thing proven to reduce the dura-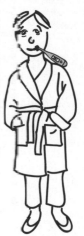tion of a cold. Let them melt in your mouth; they won't be of any use if you chew and swallow them. The zinc needs to be absorbed by your oral blood vessels. Shoot for 75 milligrams a day—roughly one lozenge every few hours. And drink warm liquids such as herbal teas or water with honey and lemon. The sweetness and acidity can stimulate salivation to clear your throat and sinuses. Warm drinks soothe the mucous membranes in your nose, mouth, and throat, reducing irritation.

If you think you're coming down with the flu, call your doctor right away and ask about antiviral remedies that can help you gain the upper hand sooner rather than later.

26 Manage Chronic Conditions

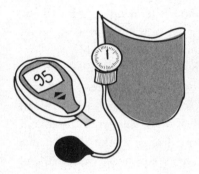

This is big. You don't want to wait until things get bad. It's so much easier to head off chronic conditions at the pass, because many are not reversible. But you can't proactively care for your body unless you undergo the blood tests and screenings appropriate for your age and history. We also have vaccines to help prevent a variety of illnesses, including ones common in later years such as shingles.

If, God forbid, you do end up having to manage something—whether temporarily or for the rest of your life—then don't slack off. Stay on top of it. This is when the severity of your condition probably dictates how well you respect its demands. For example, if you're a type-1 diabetic who relies on daily insulin just to survive, then you know you have to control your condition to a T. If you're someone with borderline type-2 diabetes whose symptoms are relatively silent, you might not be as careful, since you're not in the red zone yet. But the consequences of being so cavalier about any developing condition could be devastating, and costly.

I should add that just because we have a ton of drugs and therapies now to treat many conditions, that doesn't mean you'll want to end up having to rely on them just to live. Being drug dependent is often the result of negligence. Learn to master the management of your conditions so you help prevent or slow down their progression. In some cases, you may even be able to reverse or eliminate them entirely. Take heart from the fact that the presence of a particular condition alone can be a wonderful reminder to engage in healthy living in every area of your life, including those that have nothing to do with your illness.

27 Partner with Your Doc

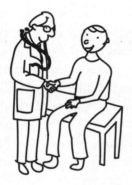

Prevention—not treatment once illness has begun—is key to optimal health and longevity. So if you haven't seen your doctor for a checkup (a quick office visit to deal with a passing cold or stomach bug doesn't count), then schedule an appointment and plan to have a comprehensive examination including any testing, vaccinations, and screenings that are relevant given your age and history.

The knowledge you bring to your doctor is more essential than your doctor's knowledge. Unfortunately, the economics of twenty-first-century medicine means that more and more physicians spend less and less time with patients. It's up to you to maximize that time. Don't assume your doctor is going to ask you every possible question to arrive at every potential solution to your concerns now and in the future. Many signs and symptoms you experience can be noted by you before you reach the doctor's office. Some people pay attention to every detail of their stock portfolio on a daily basis but not to themselves. Why not? We want quick fixes, I know. We are overloaded with information. We can feel so overwhelmed by our obligations and commitments that we end up wanting to trust someone else to make our health decisions, such as our doctor. But I'm here to tell you, this won't keep you on the best path to health.

I also recommend that you bring a friend or family member with you when you visit the doctor. It creates more accountability; you also have another set of ears. Many of us aren't in an ideal frame of mind when we're in the doctor's office, especially when something is wrong, so having someone else there can make the whole visit more bearable—and you'll remember details that you might otherwise forget. Alternatively, bring a device that can record what you hear. Many smart phones today come with a recording feature, or you can download an app to turn your phone into a voice recorder.

Modern medicine is finally moving away from the traditional "doctor knows best" paternalistic mode of decision making, in which health-care providers make key decisions for their patients. This type of decision making is slowly giving way to what we call "informed choice" or "shared decision making," in which the patient makes the final decision based on his or her goals, value system, and tolerance for risk.

A lot of decisions made in medicine today are based on someone's value system, so be sure that your opinions and convictions are respected. There's rarely a single "right" decision for treating a particular stage in a disease. The right decision for you will be the one you and your doctor arrive at together, whether it entails observation, drugs, surgery, or a combination thereof. So if you cannot speak candidly and comfortably with your doctor, find another doctor.

28 Strengthen Your Core and Maintain Good Posture

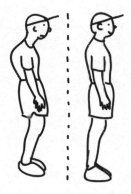

You can tell a lot about someone just by looking at the way he carries himself. Is he hunched over like an old person? Does he slouch with his head down as if he is depressed? Or is he walking fully erect, chest up, as if he is ready to take on the world with a smile on his face? With the right posture, anyone can appear younger, thinner, and more confident. But these effects aren't just for vanity's sake. Maintaining correct posture may be one of the best-kept secrets for achieving a longer, healthier, and more enjoyable life. We know that poor posture can lead to a wide assortment of neck and back problems. It is often caused by a weak core, which is one of the primary risk factors for back problems—at every age. Poor posture can also cause headaches, TMJ, arthritis, poor circulation, muscle aches, difficulty breathing, indigestion, constipation, joint stiffness, fatigue, neurological problems, and poor physical function in general.

But the risks don't end there. It's well documented that people with what's called hyperkyphosis—a posture that's hunched over, with the head and shoulders rolled forward—are 2 times more likely to die from pulmonary problems and 2.4 times more likely to die from atherosclerosis (a disorder characterized by a narrowing and hardening of the arteries due to plaque buildup) than those with normal posture. What's more, these individuals are 1.44 times more likely to die of any cause than those with healthy posture. Even people with a mild degree of hyperkyphosis are likely to die sooner.

Bear in mind that posture also plays into our emotional state. Because posture is often linked to our facial expressions, it can subconsciously drive our emotions: when we stand tall and erect, we exude confidence. This in turn helps us to feel good about ourselves and have an optimistic outlook. All roads to perfect posture start with a sturdy core. You don't need a chiseled six-pack, but engage in exercises that work this area.

29 Smile

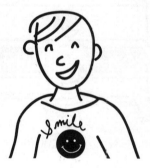

(Hint: Smiling will boost your mood no matter what. The act itself will trigger the release of pain-killing, brain-happy endorphins and serotonin. Besides, it's easier to smile; it takes seventeen muscles to smile and forty-three to frown.)

Maybe laugh a little, too.

30 Pursue Your Passions

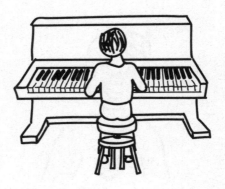

In college, I was a rower. More recently (several years beyond twenty-something), I've picked up tennis, horseback riding, and yoga. I love switching my hobbies around as I age so that I keep myself enthusiastically in the game while I also honor my body's changes through the decades. A lot of my hobbies today revolve around my kids, and my pursuits will continue to evolve as they grow older and I, of course, experience changes with the passage of time. It's important that we all develop hobbies that fulfill us in many ways—from the body's physical needs to move and play to our emotional needs to connect with other people and enjoy sports. If you were an endurance runner in your youth, you might find it hard to keep that up as you reach middle age, and you would do well to take up a new sport that's far less abusive to your knees and joints. The key is not to give up. Find a new hobby, or start learning to play an instrument, cook, garden, or pursue another passion that affords you the same rewards and will last for a while. Just be sure to choose activities that won't be abandoned quickly or that aren't highly impractical. Rather than trying to become a skydiver at seventy, for instance, check out your local Pilates studio or join a dance class at your community rec center.

31 Be Positive

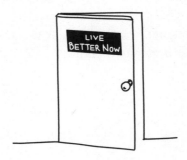

I'm a firm believer that hope and optimism are powerful forces in our lives. As with so many things, how we think determines what we experience—good or bad. And nowhere is this truer than with our health. Whether or not we have faith in our health has everything to do with whether or not we have a healthy body. If we believe we can be healthier, guess what: we will be.

Some of the most dramatic experiments putting this idea to the test are those in which people unknowingly receive fake (placebo) treatments for real health problems and come out reporting that they have improved just as much as those who got the real treatment. The placebo effect is all about a positive belief system. On the other side of the equation are stories that reveal the power of a negative belief system, one of which was famously documented in 1974 when Sam Londe was diagnosed with esophageal cancer. At the time such a diagnosis was a death sentence, so no one was surprised when he died a few weeks later, despite treatment. But what shocked the medical community was the discovery upon autopsy that Sam didn't have esophageal cancer at all. Did *thinking* that he had terminal cancer cause his premature death?

Whether or not that legendary story is in fact true down to every detail is still up for debate, but it's similar to other anecdotal evidence pointing to the power of thought. I myself notice a dramatic difference in patients' prognoses between those who believe in themselves and those who don't. In general, people who approach their life optimistically do better in clinical trials. If you believe that you are on the decline and will suffer and soon die, you may very well become a victim of such a self-fulfilling prophecy. By the same token, if you believe that you can beat the odds and enjoy a long life, you just might.

There are many ways you can boost your positive outlook. Organized, deistic religions can achieve this, but so can secular belief systems. All you need is a system that helps you to put even indescribable suffering into a wider context and tap into a higher awareness of yourself. Such a system also facilitates your sense of community and connection to other people, which is healing in itself.

32 Find Out What Exercise or Activity You're Bad at and Focus on It

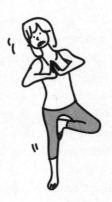

There is always room for improvement. I'm not asking you to force yourself to do anything that you truly loathe or that is completely unmotivating, but you'd be surprised by what you can discover if you try something outside your normal comfort zone. This will simultaneously challenge your body and brain in ways that can be healthful. We tend to stick with activities that we're used to doing, and that the body is well conditioned to handle. But new challenges can make us mentally sharper and physically fitter. When we push ourselves to engage in activities that we're not used to, we effectively force our brains to think harder and we compel our bodies to adapt to different circumstances. Bad at swimming? Hit the pool and see if you can swim a few laps today, more tomorrow. This will stimulate your body and work latent muscles that are hungry for action. Never cooked a meal from scratch for a party of ten? Sign up for a cooking class. This will tap creative areas of your brain that you haven't flexed in a while. Can't touch your toes or balance on one foot? Focus on stretching more (and see Rule 44) and work on your balance. You'll need that flexibility and sense of balance the older you get to keep up with normal activities. By identifying activities that you're bad at, you can improve your body's weak spots and at the same time find fun, engaging hobbies that you may grow to love.

33 Protect Your Eyes and Ears

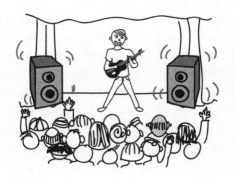

Most of us take our senses for granted if they are alive and well. But we don't realize how much our quality of life hinges on those senses—being able to hear, touch, taste, smell, and see. And many of us have at least one or two senses in particular from which we derive a lot of pleasure and/or profit. Think of the surgeon who needs his eyesight and sense of touch to execute his skill. Or the chef who relies on her sense of taste and smell to craft award-winning meals. The composer who depends on his ears to hear the notes and his hands to feel the instrument he plays. Losing your senses is not necessarily inevitable if you protect them over time and keep track of any changes so you can discuss them with your doctor. This is especially true when it comes to your eyes and ears—two senses that can be directly impacted by the way you choose live.

While we can't do anything about the loud rock concerts we attended in our youth or the days we didn't wear sunglasses while outside, we can do better going forward. Do you watch the volume on your headphones as you listen to music? Do you protect your eyes while enjoying the sun? The longer you can keep your eyes clear and your ears sensitive to sound, the longer you can enjoy seeing and hearing without medical intervention.

34 Don't Forget Your Teeth and Feet

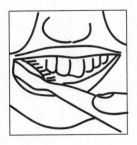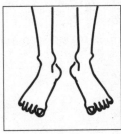

Many years ago, some researchers claimed that gum disease could lead to heart disease. While the two may not sound related, scientists believe that the heart can be weakened by agents in the blood that respond to inflammation, and chronic gum disease produces constant inflammation. So flossing at least once a day is a good idea. Not only will it go a long way toward protecting your teeth and gums (and lowering your body's overall inflammation), it's also just plain old good hygiene.

There's no serious science to prove that one of the biggest regrets of older folks is that they failed to take care of their teeth and feet when they were young. But large surveys and personal accounts from people who spend a lot of time with the elderly tell us this is so. If allowed to deteriorate, teeth and feet will cause misery. Poor oral hygiene can produce terrible tooth decay or, worse, the total loss of teeth; not taking care of your feet can result in painful bunions, corns, warts, and other podiatric torments that make walking difficult, if not impossible. What's more, the feet contain thousands of receptors that help you to gain information about your whereabouts—literally. Many of these receptors contribute to your sense of balance and ability to walk. A whopping one-quarter of the bones in the body are located in the feet, demonstrating their complexity. And let's not forget that together, our teeth and feet are major connectors to the world around us. We use our teeth to obtain nourishment and our feet to navigate our paths through life.

So don't forget them. Visit the dentist at least once a year, twice if you've got a mouth prone to problems (your dentist can tell you that—he or she is a partner in your health care, too). Ask about proper brushing, flossing, and which toothpaste and toothbrush are best to use (and don't forget to tend to the health and hygiene of your tongue— the only muscle in the body that's attached at one end). The newer electronic toothbrushes might be worth the extra money if they prevent you from long, expensive stays in the dentist's chair getting uncomfortable dental work done.

As for your feet, splurge on foot massages once in a while if that's your thing. Take note of weird-looking or painful growths or discolorations that emerge and do something about them. Buy good and comfortable shoes! Trust me, your teeth and feet will thank you later on.

35 Learn CPR

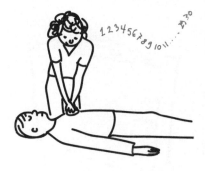

I won't teach you this lifesaving skill here, but learn it. The American Heart Association and lots of community centers conduct classes throughout the year. Sign up and get certified. You never know when you might need to use it. Best of all: most courses today (and they will take up only half a Saturday morning, if that) will teach you how to use a defibrillator, how to deal with a choking incident, and how to revive an infant who stops breathing—all excellent skills to have that don't require rigorous study, training, or even a test!

36 Make a Mobile Supply Kit for Emergencies

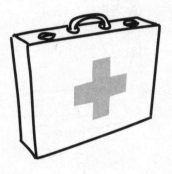

Disasters can strike at any time, anywhere. From wild weather patterns that prompt tornadoes, hurricanes, and blizzards to earthquakes, tsunamis, nuclear fallouts, and dark days like 9/11, unexpected catastrophes can be buffered by preparation. Being ready will also help you to survive a disaster and recover sooner. Have a plan with family members about where to meet if a catastrophe strikes and how to get in touch with one another (remember, your cell phone might not work, and if you don't have a way to recharge it, it may not last long).

Sites like Ready.gov can give you plenty of tips on how to prepare, including making a disaster kit. Below are some essentials you'll want to put together, as suggested by the Federal Emergency Management Agency*

- One gallon of water per person per day for at least three days, for drinking and sanitation
- At least a three-day supply of nonperishable food
- Battery-powered or hand-crank radio, a NOAA weather radio with tone alert, and extra batteries
- Flashlight and extra batteries
- First aid kit
- Whistle to signal for help
- Dust mask to help filter contaminated air and plastic sheeting and duct tape to shelter in place
- Moist towelettes, garbage bags, and plastic ties for personal sanitation
- Wrenches or pliers to turn off utilities
- Manual can opener for food
- Local maps
- Cell phone with charger, inverter, or solar charger

---

* Adapted from the Federal Emergency Management Agency's list at www .fema.gov.

Additional items to consider given your circumstances:

- Prescription medications (a full week's supply) and glasses or contact lenses
- Infant formula and diapers
- Pet food and extra water for your pets
- Cash or traveler's checks and change
- Important family documents such as copies of insurance policies, identification, and bank account records in a waterproof, portable container
- Sleeping bag or warm blanket for each person. Consider additional bedding if you live in a cold climate.
- Complete change of clothing, including a long-sleeved shirt, long pants, and sturdy shoes. Consider additional clothing if you live in a cold climate.
- Household chlorine bleach and a medicine dropper. When diluted to nine parts water to one part bleach, bleach can be used as a disinfectant. Or in an emergency, you can use it to treat drinking water by using sixteen drops of regular household liquid bleach per gallon of water. Do not use scented or color safe bleach, or bleaches with added cleaners, to treat drinking water.
- Fire extinguisher
- Matches in a waterproof container
- Feminine supplies and personal hygiene items
- Mess kits, paper cups, plates, paper towels, and plastic utensils

- Paper and pencils or pens
- Books, games, puzzles, or other activities for children

And while you're at it, throw in a copy of *The Worst-Case Scenario Survival Handbook* by Joshua Piven. That should answer any lingering questions you have when a crisis comes. Store all your emergency supplies in waterproof containers that are easy to access.

37 Eat More Than Three Servings of Cold-Water Fish a Week

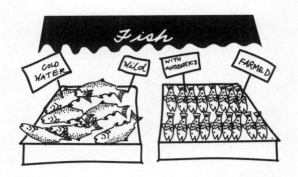

Cold-water fish, such as salmon, sardines, tuna, trout, anchovies, herring, halibut, cod, black cod, mackerel, and mahi-mahi are excellent sources of high-quality protein, healthy fats, and naturally occurring vitamins and minerals. Aim to eat cold-water fish a minimum of three times per week. The one exception: it's better to avoid fish than to consume any sea creatures that are not recommended by Seafood Watch,* which keeps a running record of safe, ocean-friendly seafood. You'll want to skip fish high in mercury and anything from dirty waters. Wherever possible, buy wild-caught fish.

---

* For details relating to where you live, refer to http://www.montereybay aquarium.org/cr/cr_seafoodwatch/download.aspx.

38 Eat at Least Five Servings of Fruits and Vegetables a Day

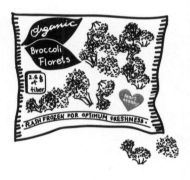

There is convincing evidence that eating at least five servings of fruits and vegetables a day can help prevent chronic diseases, not to mention decrease one's risk for obesity. But most people consume less than two cups of fruits and veggies a day, far below the four to six cups we should be getting. Think of it this way: the more fruits and veggies you consume, the less likely you'll be to replace them with nutrient-poor, health-depleting options. So eat up, and if you're going to favor one type of produce over the other, go for more leafy greens and fibrous vegetables than sugary fruit. Choose many colors, as nature segregates nutrients by color; the blend of nutrients that makes a carrot orange is different from the blend that makes broccoli green, but they both are needed to support health. To maximize the number of different nutrients you consume, you're better off eating a yellow bell pepper and a red one than eating two of a single color. Flash-frozen is fine and may actually be better than fresh (see Rule 5).

39 Speak Strongly to the Next Generation

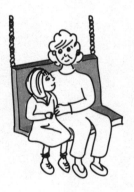

It's quite natural to feel invincible when you're young and to shun any recommendations about how to be healthy. But when you're young, you're setting the foundation for your later years. So as adults, it's important that we do our best to inform and teach the next generation. The key is to find words and images that are relevant to them. Find a way to explain things to young people so that they can understand your vocabulary and jargon. While I was teaching a lesson on antioxidants to a lay audience, someone recommended that I use different colored marbles to represent types of free radicals in the body. At the time I thought it was rather goofy, but it worked. Visual imagery can be powerful and convincing especially to younger folks.

I once had a tough time telling my kids why chocolate milk isn't the best thing for them. It wasn't until I showed them a demonstration marvelously performed by celebrity chef Jamie Oliver that they finally understood me (and heeded my advice). Jamie put sugar consumption into dramatic perspective when he filled a yellow school bus with the amount of sugar added to the Los Angeles Unified School District's flavored milk in one week. It was a visually overwhelming scene to watch as the "sugar" (in this case, white sand) rose above the windows and overtook the bus.

Some parents find it easier to talk about sex than to discuss issues with food that could touch on matters of weight or weight-related diseases like anorexia. But the sooner you establish an open communication pattern, the sooner your kids will come back to ask more questions and, believe it or not, ask for your advice. Remember, they won't accept any sage words of wisdom from an elder unless they can comprehend what's in it for them and how it will affect them. They will want to know, Why does it matter to me now? When my kids understood just how much sugar they consume thanks to Mr. Oliver's visual example, they still wanted to know why it mattered to them at that moment. That's when I had to explain that their eating habits play into how well they perform—at school and in sports. If they want to be able to think clearly, ace exams, and win important games for their team, they need to be mindful of how they are nourishing their brains and bodies. It's not always easy to make certain facts highly relevant to kids, but when you relate things to their current goals and ambitions, you have a better chance of getting them to listen.

40 Embrace Your OCD Side

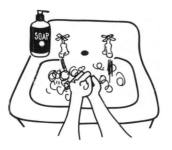

A little bit of obsessive-compulsive disorder can go a long way to keeping you healthy. You don't need to alphabetize your medicine cabinet, accumulate junk, or wear white gloves when you drive, but if you consider what OCD offers—reliable routines—you can see how it might relate to staying healthy. With a little OCD, you'll remember to wash your hands regularly, especially after exposure to germy things like bathrooms and raw chicken. You'll be strict with your daily schedule. And you'll maintain tidy living quarters that will help with your hygiene and peace of mind.

41 Never Skip Breakfast

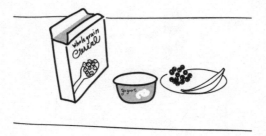

This old adage will never die. After fasting all night long, your body needs a metabolic jump-start to begin the day. We know that people who eat breakfast are just plain healthier in general and rarely have issues with weight (and if they do, the weight sloughs off once they start eating breakfast!). Skipping those morning calories to lose weight is one of the worst habits a person can develop. Front-loading your eating in the early part of the day will prevent you from overconsuming later, help you burn more calories, and allow you to get a wallop of nutrients when you need them. Moreover, eating breakfast will give your brain a much-needed boost, fueling your productivity and creativity for the entire day. If you wait too long to eat after rising, stress hormones will start pumping and sabotage your body's healthy metabolism. Too high a concentration of stress hormones like cortisol will encourage your body to retain fat, among other undesirable things.

42 Seventeen Milligrams Twice a Day

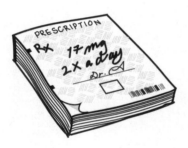

This rule is wholly mine. Whenever someone asks me to prescribe *something* to make her feel better, I often joke, "Seventeen milligrams twice a day." It's my way of saying there is no cure-all or pill that will make you feel better. You hear about people getting vitamin B_{12} shots or vitamin infusions and they miraculously improve. The path to improvement is not finding the one thing you are lacking—it's following a collection of rules. By sticking to as many as possible, your chance of a long, fulfilling life goes up.

43 Take the Positive from Getting a Disease

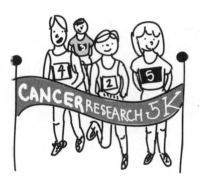

Don't throw out the rules of prevention once you've been diagnosed with an illness or medical condition. Consider such a diagnosis a wake-up call. Use the opportunity to focus on yourself and develop more long-term health strategies. Having heart disease, for instance, doesn't give you permission to eat red meat five days a week and skip exercise. Neither does it mean you earn a free pass to avoid the things you can do to prevent *other* health challenges likely brewing beneath the surface. Cancer doctors like me know that most patients who survive their cancer don't actually die of cancer in the end. They succumb to something else, usually as a result of neglecting that area of their life as they focused too much on their cancer. For example, women who survive breast cancer are more likely to die of heart disease than of cancer. So don't forget the general rules of prevention while you're managing a condition or combating a particular illness.

44 S-T-R-E-T-C-H

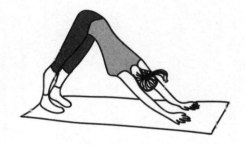

You don't have to aspire to an Olympic gymnast's flexibility, but make room for stretching exercises in your routine. This will help you to maintain the physical pliancy you need to keep up with normal day-to-day activities like getting in and out of cars, navigating your kitchen, and picking up objects. It also will help you to work on two other key skills: coordination and balance. According to the U.S. Centers for Disease Control and Prevention, one of every three Americans over the age of sixty-five falls each year, and among individuals aged sixty-five to eighty-four, falls account for 87 percent of all fractures and are the second leading cause of spinal cord and brain injury.

So in addition to your physical activities, make room for stretching. Your joints—and your inner yogi—will love it.

45 Keep a To-Do List

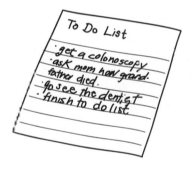

To Do List

· get a colonoscopy
· ask mom how grand-
  father died.
· go see the dentist
· finish to do list

Lists are great for many things beyond shopping. They are an automatic scorecard, a way to track ourselves, and a means to hold ourselves accountable for what we want to achieve. Alongside your one-, five-, ten-, and twenty-year plans, keep a to-do list that contains those little steps and strategies that you're tackling. To-do lists can be created for all sorts of major goals, so don't limit yourself to just one long list. Maintain daily, weekly, and yearly lists. Daily to-do lists can contain your top priorities for the day, the minutes you want to spend in motion, the time you've blocked off to take a breather, and your bedtime. Weekly to-do lists might spell out the meals you want to cook, friends you want to catch up with, and the hobby you want to try or your new ideas for a workout routine. Yearly lists should include reminders for doctor visits, screening tests, and annual vaccines.

If you share your big-goal lists with family members you can count on the good ol' accountability factor to keep you motivated.

46 Ask for Help

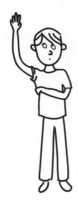

It takes a lot of courage to ask for help. We are incredibly autonomous creatures, and as Americans we especially are inclined to act independently. We prefer to solve problems on our own and value stubbornness as if it were a positive characteristic. But sometimes our challenges are just too big. Know where your limitations are, and respect them. There is nothing wrong with asking for help when the time comes, whether it's asking for support in learning how to live with diabetes, getting to the bottom of your insomnia, designing a dietary and exercise protocol that suits your needs, or finding a therapist to deal with psychological issues that are affecting your quality of life. Don't assume you can take care of everything all the time. None of us can. And none of us can be an expert in everything, even with the Internet at our fingertips. Be willing to surrender and enjoy the benefits of someone else's wisdom and experience—from professionals to friends, who can take the stress out of a concern or worry by sharing their own struggles.

47 Have Children

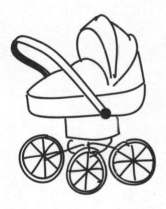

This rule won't be for everyone, but here's one reason why it's worth entertaining the idea: you'd be more likely to live longer than your childless counterparts. Seems counter-intuitive because with children comes a lot of extra stress. But perhaps part of the reason people who have kids outlive those who don't is that they take better care of themselves in general and are less likely to engage in the kinds of activities that increase their risk for premature death. There's also something to be said for all that running around you do with children. The mere act of raising a child compels us to remain active and mentally challenged—both good things for health.

48 Comply

Being able to prevent, manage, and treat any condition or illness successfully hinges on being able to comply with recommended medications, including dosage (how much to take) and timing (when it's best to take it). Noncompliance is one of the biggest problems in health care today; according to a 2005 Harris Interactive report, roughly half of all prescriptions for drugs to be taken on an ongoing basis are either not completed or are never filled in the first place. Drugs that treat asymptomatic conditions, such as high blood pressure or high cholesterol, are the most likely not to be taken. Yet in the long term, the effects of not taking these medications can be devastating. The lesson: regardless of how you feel, abide by your medication's instructions as if your life depended on it, and if you don't, be honest about it with your doctor.

49 Pick Up a Pooch

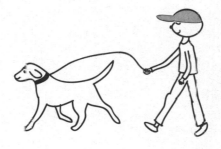

It's long been known anecdotally that dog owners are often the happiest, most upbeat people. But it's not all about the companionship of having a pooch to love and care for. Owning a dog demands that you maintain a relatively constant and reliable timetable, tending to the animal's ritualistic feedings, walks, and naps. In other words, it has the overall effect of forcing set patterns that foster health—namely sticking to a regular schedule. It also helps that walking a dog compels you to move, to engage in at least some physical exercise, even if Fido isn't a feisty greyhound looking for a run. Being outside in nature with dogs also offers the benefits of downtime, as walking dogs requires that you leave your desk and cease multitasking—other than scooping up poop and talking on your cell phone at the same time.

50 Have the Toughest Conversation

Sorry to bring you down, but this rule is typically swept under the proverbial rug until after the fact. Conversations about end-of-life decisions and life-sustaining medical treatment are not fun. But they make for far easier moments when the time comes to deal with a family crisis. There is no enjoyment in meeting doctors for the first time and coping with complex medical issues you have never encountered (or that your loved ones face when you're incapacitated). Should you become incapacitated and doctors turn to your family members for answers, they should be prepared for questions like, Do you want everything possible done to keep you alive? Nothing? If you have to go on life support, is that okay with you? Where do you want to draw the line? Who is responsible for making decisions on your behalf? Although we'd hope that our family members can agree on making decisions based on our wishes, unless things are spelled out somewhere (in a legal document such as a living will or health proxy), arguments and discord can arise quickly. So prevent that from ever happening by having a set of nonnegotiable instructions that leaves no room for doubt or disagreement.

A number of tools are available today to guide you through conveying your wishes under a worst-case scenario. A good place to start is the Prepare website (prepareforyour care.org), designed by researchers from the San Francisco VA Medical Center and the University of California, San Francisco.

51 | Understand Basic Biovocabulary

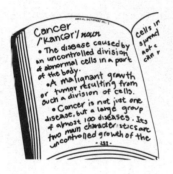

Could you define "inflammation" in a sentence or two? Do you know what "cancer" really is? How about "heart disease" and the signs of a heart attack? Do you know the difference between a "vitamin" and a "medication"? Or, for that matter, a "drug" and a "supplement"?

These are key terms everyone should understand; they crop up every day in the popular media. Read up on them so that when you come across health headlines in the news, you can understand what the article is saying and how the new research might apply to you. Think of it this way: When you shop for a car, you're knowledgeable about important lingo like what "zero to sixty" means, or how highway MPG differs from city MPG. Knowing certain definitions in the car industry allows you to make better decisions about which car to buy. The same holds true in the health industry. When you're familiar with fundamental vocabulary, you're empowered to make better decisions about your health.

52 Make Your Own Definition of Health

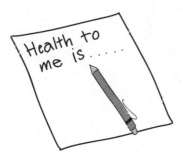

What does being healthy mean to you? Running a mile in under six minutes? Looking svelte enough to adorn the cover of a magazine? Having control of your diabetes? Avoiding the ills of your parents and living until one hundred? Everyone's definition will be different. Figure out what your personal definition of health is, and from there, develop your own code of health—the rules you'll abide by to live up to that definition.

This entails coming up with your own set of data points, rules, or standards that say something about your health. Your weight, for instance, could be a personal metric. Your need to eat dinner by 7:00 p.m. and go to bed at exactly 9:30 p.m. to feel good the next day is also a metric. From a broader perspective, you can look at metrics as a set of habits or customs that either enhance or detract from your health.

I've given you a lot of potential metrics by which to measure your health in this part of the book. Now we'll turn to the things you would do well to avoid.

PART II

What to Avoid

53 Bad Ingredients and Fad Diets

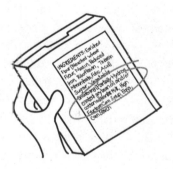

Trans fats. High-fructose corn syrup. Preservatives. Food colorings. Flavorings. Additives. MSG. Texturizers. Artificial sweeteners. Hydrolized protein. Ammonia. Fruit juice concentrate. Sodium on steroids. You know these ingredients won't win you an award for having a clean diet. Nor will foods that are known by trademarked names around the world, like Whopper, Yoplait, Cheez-It, Coke, Cinnabon,

Lucky Charms, and so on. As with anything, they are fine in moderation. Remember Rule 5: Eat real food (most of the time). Real food doesn't come with a list of ingredients or claims about what it can do for you. Real food doesn't have a long shelf life and will do what living things do once they are cut from their roots or killed: it will rot.

But what about things like gluten, soy, and GMO (genetically modified organisms) that have gotten a bad rap lately? Without a doubt many people suffer from food intolerances and sensitivities and should steer clear of those ingredients that irritate their digestive systems or otherwise wreak havoc on their bodies. In large quantities, soy can disrupt the hormonal system, so moderate your consumption of it (and for the record: fermented soy that's ubiquitous in Asian cuisine is not the same as the nonfermented soy protein that is everywhere in the Western food supply). But if you eat primarily real foods, you need to worry much less about these taboo ingredients, or any others for that matter. You won't consume them in the amounts that can cause harm. Remember, too, that even products labeled "gluten free" are usually just that—products. They aren't real food.

As for GMO? Rest assured, genetically modified foods won't kill you either. GMO corn won't cause cancer, but the stress you endure while you worry about it will raise your risk. (Tidbit: We owe a lot of the hysteria around GMO to British environmentalist Mark Lynas, who was at the heart of the anti-GMO movement. In January 2013, Mr. Lynas changed his mind completely and is now a staunch GMO advocate. Why? In his words: "Well, the answer is fairly simple: I discovered science, and in the process I hope I became a better environmentalist." Amen to that.)

Speaking of science, be careful about diets that promise to cure you of everything or that have you doing weird things like taking detox supplements or undergoing liver cleanses (see the next rule). The vast majority of these diets are not backed by any scientific data and are purely profit driven. Their promoters employ lots of pseudoscience and conspiracy theories to push their agenda (and products). To some degree, diets can be helpful if they guide you to better-quality foods and teach you principles of portion control and nutrition. But there's a lot of noise out there in the diet world that tries to trump common sense and gut instinct—literally. I trust you know the difference between an apple and an apple fritter. And the great divide between a gluten-free soy burger with processed American cheese and a sirloin burger with portobello mushrooms. Which burger was made from ingredients you can actually visualize?

54 Detoxes

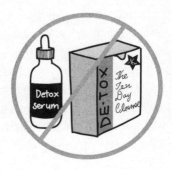

Your body is expertly designed to detox naturally thanks to your kidneys, liver, sweat glands, lungs, and digestive system. You don't need to take drastic, sometimes dangerous, measures to detoxify your body, and this includes the use of supplements and detox formulas marketed to clean you out. They are nonsense. Many of these protocols have few or no studies to back up their overpromising claims, which include reducing or removing toxins, cleansing the colon, purifying the blood, spurring weight loss, flushing fat, and treating disease. Some can be downright scary—not to mention perilous for the body. Before you even consider embarking on one of these regimes, insist on randomized studies that show these agents will produce a meaningful result. In the meantime, don't experiment on yourself before the real proof is available and widely accepted by the medical community.

We do live in a more polluted world now, but we need to be careful about accepting brash, extreme statements about the connection between toxins and possible impacts. I should point out that one of the longest-living communities on Earth—where a remarkable number of people live past one hundred—is tucked behind smoggy Los Angeles in Loma Linda. Toxins will accumulate in your body over time; it's as inevitable as the wrinkles that you'll get and the gray hair you'll grow. But there's no safe way to remove them other than relying on the body's built-in systems, which are well equipped to handle the job.

And there's no such thing as an "immune-boosting" anything. The best way to enhance your immune system is to eat well and stay active. Superfoods don't exist, either. Yes, some foods contain more nutrients than others, but it's quite hyperbolic and misleading to call any food a "superfood." Don't be fooled by anyone selling you something to "oxygenate" your body. Your lungs do that for you. Watch out for the word "cleansing," too. Your body has built-in mechanisms for that. The only things we should be cleansing are our skin, hair, teeth, and probably our garages.

55 Risky Behaviors and Dangerous Sports

We'd like to avoid trauma as much as possible, not just for ourselves but also for our family members. Injury yields damage that tends to last a long time, if not forever. So it pays to ask yourself where and when you're willing to take risks that could have life-altering consequences.

Have you ever played or do you currently play a contact sport such as football, ice hockey, soccer, rugby, lacrosse, water polo, wrestling, boxing, or basketball? Do your kids? Contact sports don't just put you at risk for short-term injuries such as cuts, bruises, bone fractures, and pulled muscles, tendons, and ligaments. Repeated injuries, especially trauma to the head even when it doesn't cause a concussion, will have a lasting impact due to the inflammatory reactions that take place in the brain and body. This explains why so many NFL players suffer from premature heart disease and stroke while nuns win the longevity contest. It also may shed light on the shocking number of suicides among those who've suffered repeated blows to the head in contact sports, but who would not otherwise seem to be at risk of killing themselves.

Similarly, any risky behavior could shorten your life and the quality of it. These include the obvious things like smoking or drinking and driving, and they also include the not-so-obvious things like trying a triple-diamond ski run when you're a beginner or running a marathon without training. I think you know what I mean. It's one thing to challenge yourself once in a while and do something outside your normal comfort zone. But it's another thing to make a habit of thrill seeking and engaging in risky behaviors that have very obvious and known dangers. Life insurance companies don't ask you if you scuba dive or pilot a small airplane for nothing.

56 Airport Backscatter X-ray Scanners

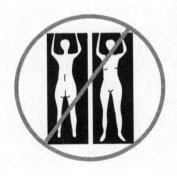

Do we really know what these machines do to us? Where's the long-term data going back decades to show they are indeed harmless? In the 1930s and '40s, shoe fitters used a type of X-ray machine called a fluoroscope to take pictures of people's feet. And guess what: those who were exposed to excessive radiation went on to develop cancers on their feet.

So until science can prove the safety of backscatter technology, I'll be requesting the manual pat-down massage when I go through the TSA's gateway at airports. You should, too. And let's campaign for better technology that doesn't entail shooting radiation through someone. (As an aside, we may be seeing these scanners gone from our airports due to all the controversy they've generated, but be aware of similar technologies that emerge without a bona fide safety history.)

57 Sunburns

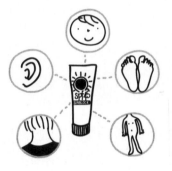

Your skin weighs approximately twice as much as your brain. It's a huge organ that acts as a barrier to protect your insides. But the fairer you are, the higher your risk for blistering sunburns. While the symptoms of sunburn are usually temporary, the skin damage is often permanent and can have serious long-term health effects, including premature aging and skin cancer. Although you shed and regrow your outer skin cells about every twenty-seven days, injury that lies hidden deep inside can manifest years later. The experience of getting a sunburn is also a lesson in inflammation, which can have a lasting impact on the body long after the burn is gone. You don't need to get a sunburn to absorb enough rays to create vitamin D, but you do need to protect your skin from the harmful effects of ultraviolet radiation. Don't forget about those hard-to-reach places such as the tops of your ears, back of your neck, and scalp (opt for a hat in that case).

5 8 Insomnia

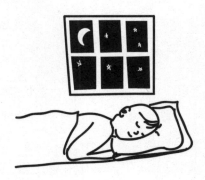

Bad nights make for bad days. We all know what lack of sleep does to us. It makes us moody, mentally foggy, unproductive, uncreative, insufferably tired, and oddly uncoordinated (some argue that serious lack of sleep is on par with drunkenness in terms of what it does to our motor skills). But those are just the obvious symptoms you probably notice. What you don't necessarily see is what's going on from a biochemical standpoint. Suffice it to say that sleep deprivation is a villain to well-being, and its antidote—restful sleep—is an unsung hero in our world. Among its proven effects, sleep can dictate how much we eat, how fat we get, whether we can fight off infections, how creative and insightful we can be, how much we can remember, how well we can learn new things, how easily we can cope with stress, and how fast we can process information. The brain is much more active at night than during the day. If you lose just one and a half hours that your body needs for one night, your daytime alertness will go down by about a third. In fact, we can make do longer without food than without sleep. The side effects of poor sleep habits are many: hypertension, confusion, memory loss, the inability to acquire new knowledge, obesity, cardiovascular disease, and depression. And when we consider the parallels between our obesity epidemic and collective sleep deprivation, we have to wonder: could sleep be the ultimate diet?

Sixty-five percent of Americans are overweight or obese, a percentage that takes on a special significance when an estimated 63 percent of American adults do not get the recommended 8 hours of sleep a night. The average adult gets 6.9 hours of sleep on weeknights and 7.5 hours on weekends, for a daily average of 7 hours. How much are you getting? Do you have fewer than 1,460 dreams a year, the average for someone who sleeps well?

For far too many people in the modern era, sleep deprivation is a badge of honor. That's why one of the first questions I ask patients who are afraid of a fatal diagnosis is simply the following: How are you sleeping?

It's no surprise that our lack of sleep has spurred an explosion in the sleep-aid industry. At least 20 percent of older American adults use some form of sleep aid, including prescription or over-the-counter drugs or even alcohol. Many use such aids every night to make them drowsy. Is taking something for sleep okay? A better question: Is this what we've come to need in contemporary society because we can't rely on our innate sleep mechanism? (And sleep is, by the way, a very natural process, like anything else our bodies do automatically for survival.)

The vast majority of people who suffer from insomnia or wakefulness during the night could find automatic, dreamy sleep again—without aids—if they identified the culprit and established a few habits to encourage 100 percent natural sleep. This means being mindful of ingredients such as caffeine that antagonize sleep if consumed too late in the day, being able to manage chronic worrisome thoughts, and being religious about going to bed at the same time every night and getting up at the same time every morning. An ideal environment for sleep is also important (for instance, no stimulating electronics in the bedroom; many of these devices emit what's called a blue light wave that will trigger wakefulness in your brain). Find a way to use sleep aids sparingly and save them for extreme circumstances such as when traveling across time zones. You may even want to take a look at which type of sleep setting is ideal for you. Are you better off in a separate bed from your spouse? Are you still trying to share a queen bed with your restless partner (who also snores)? By the age of sixty, 60 percent of men and

40 percent of women will snore during sleep. What disrupts your sleep? The number of couples choosing to sleep in separate beds or even separate rooms (upwards of 30 percent of us) isn't all that unbelievable. If you get a great night's sleep regularly, everything in life seems better, including your relationships. If you're not sleeping, there's probably a reason. Get to the bottom of it and get back those Z's. You need them.

59 Stilettos and Other Sneaky Sources of Inflammation

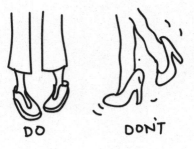

DO   DON'T

Inflammation is a normal but sometimes overactive biological response to harmful stimuli. Its ultimate goal is to initiate healing, but when inflammation becomes chronic due to disease or prolonged stress, it can become destructive. For this reason, inflammation has been linked to some of our most troubling degenerative diseases today, including heart disease, Alzheimer's disease, cancer, autoimmune diseases, diabetes, and accelerated aging.

When you're walking around barefoot or wearing uncomfortable shoes, you're causing some unnecessary inflammation in your feet that can have an impact on your entire system. If the goal is to reduce your overall inflammation and take the load off your joints and lower back to further reduce inflammation, then I know of no better, easier way to do this than to simply wear a pair of supportive and comfortable shoes daily.

Other ways to reduce sneaky sources of inflammation include maintaining a healthy weight (Rule 13), keeping a regular schedule (Rule 3), getting an annual flu shot (Rule 14), considering taking baby aspirin (Rule 22) and a statin (Rule 21), keeping a positive outlook (Rule 31), and managing any ongoing condition carefully and responsibly (Rule 26). If you have any obvious signs of chronic inflammation somewhere, be it acid reflux or back pain, take note of the condition and do what you can to resolve it.

60 Juicing

Don't think for a second that Jack LaLanne owed his longevity (he lived to be ninety-six years young) to his eponymous juicer. Perhaps he could have lived to one hundred if he had avoided this trend of pulverizing produce in a powerful blender and drinking up. Does the body really like consuming ten carrots all at once? Or a pound of radishes? The more important question to answer is whether the original nutrients in the fruits and vegetables, which are now contained in a tall glass of juice, are in fact the same. I think not.

For starters, oxygen is a powerful oxidant. It changes the chemistry of molecules in an instant by stealing electrons. As soon as we expose the inner flesh of a fruit or vegetable to the oxygen-rich air, guess what? We oxidize it on the spot, in a fraction of a second—especially if we subject the fruit or vegetable to the disruptive power of a blender. We change its whole makeup and the nutrition that went with it. There's a reason why Tropicana sells most of its juices in nontransparent, refrigerated containers that light and air cannot penetrate. They've been in the business a long time. They know how to preserve the nutrients in their product as long as possible.

I've already stressed the importance of eating whole real foods. Juice from a juicer is not whole food—it's *processed*, because the fiber with its phytonutrients has been removed. When people say that juicing saved their health or somehow transformed their bodies, they are really saying it distracted them from eating junk food.

While the peddlers of juice drinks like to refer to all the studies about the benefits of consuming more fresh fruits and vegetables, they fail to mention that these studies don't have anything to do with juice products. They are taken from studies done on whole foods. That's like comparing apples to oranges (excuse the pun). Which means you know what you should be doing: junking the juicer and eating whole foods.

61 Eating More Than Three Servings of Red and/or Processed Meats a Week

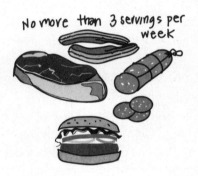

No more than 3 servings per week

As with alcohol, there are pluses and minuses to being a meat lover. The consumption of red meat in moderation isn't necessarily bad, but studies have shown that eating more than three servings a week can increase your risk for certain diseases and chronic conditions. There is also ample data that processed meats such as deli cuts, salami, ham, bacon, hot dogs, and sausages can have negative health effects. One possible explanation is that these processed meats may contain high concentrations of salt or chemicals that can be harmful. So moderate your consumption of them.

62 Vitamins and Supplements

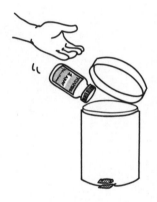

If you look at all the vitamin studies done on groups of more than a thousand people in the last few decades, many of them have shown that taking vitamin supplements is correlated with an increased risk of diseases such as cancer and produces little benefit to health. Some of these results were statistically significant, but some were not. The interactions of supplements and the body are very complex, but a simple explanation may be that the body likes to create free radicals to attack 'bad" cells, including cancerous ones. If you block that mechanism by taking copious amounts of vitamins, especially those touted as antioxidants, you block your body's natural ability to control itself. You block a physiological process You disrupt a system we don't fully understand yet.

Simply put, we cannot expect a pill or packaged food product to satisfy our nutritional needs in the same way real food can. I don't care what the label says, go for the foods that don't come with labels! And stop taking vitamins.

63 Absence of Downtime

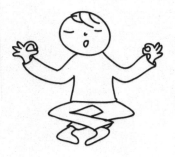

Anyone who has burned the midnight oil at work or hasn't had a restful vacation in a long time knows that a breaking point will be reached. This is when you shut down and struggle to be productive because you're just so exhausted and in need of a time-out. Too many of us try to cure our fatigue with infrequent vacations rather than scheduling downtime intermittently throughout the weeks of the year. Downtime isn't just about removing oneself from work obligations and household chores; it's also about truly relaxing in a peaceful environment in which you can let the brain take a breather and stop multitasking. This will ultimately help you to be more creative and more productive when you jump back into the game again.

Be mindful of technologies such as those found in our phones and computers, including handheld conveniences. These wondrous devices make the smallest windows of time entertaining and potentially productive. But regular use of these devices may produce an unanticipated side effect: when we keep our brains busy with digital input, we could be forfeiting downtime that could allow us to better learn and remember information, or to come up with new ideas. See if you can schedule downtime at least once or twice a week. It needn't be for long. Try a mere twenty minutes to start during which you avoid media and technology entirely and do something else pleasurable such as reading a book or going for a brisk walk (without your cell phone). Build regular downtime periods into your schedule. Your brain and body will love it.

64 Smoking

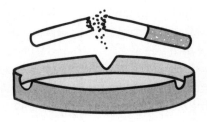

Your lungs have a lot of work to do and don't need the extra inflammation and irritation caused by tobacco. You breathe in 2,000 gallons of air a day into an organ with the surface area of a tennis court. There's enough to filter out of the air already without having to add the toxins from tobacco.

Along with being overweight, smoking is one of the most prominent risk factors in virtually all chronic illnesses. It can significantly increase your risk for all types of ailments and affect your quality of life. Anyone who quits the habit gains tremendous benefits in terms of health and longevity.

While smoking can do lasting damage, the good news is that the lungs can regenerate once you stop. And it's never too late to quit smoking.

It may be legal in some places, but just because it's okay to buy and smoke marijuana doesn't make it okay for your health. We know that marijuana use can cripple the immune system and increases the risk for respiratory illnesses, cancers, and mental disorders like depression and memory defects.

65 Hoarding Your Medical Information

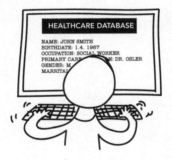

Keeping your medical information secret will do you more harm than good. You don't have to tell everyone your name, weight, cholesterol level, and what health issues you've got, but if you are given the opportunity to share your information anonymously with science (and the world at large), then do it. This will help us to build the kind of database we need to mine so we can come up with better technologies and therapies to yes, save you and your family. This isn't about privacy. It's about giving back the raw data that we need to create new opportunities for people to live longer.

Perhaps the best way to illustrate this is to consider what happened in the fall of 2008 when Google predicted a flu outbreak three weeks before the Centers for Disease Control. How? It tracked how many people were searching for words like "fever," "chill," and "flu" and where they were. This online "sharing," in turn, led to Google's early and correct prediction as millions around the world created patterns in their online searches that could be detected and identified. Imagine the power of such an early call, which helped alert and mobilize health authorities so they could get ahead of the curve.

So share and share alike. And if your employer offers an interactive corporate wellness program, sign up!

PART III

Doctor's Orders

The purpose of this section is to give you a decade-by-decade list of things to do, from the information that you should be collecting routinely about yourself to the preventive steps you can take at each age. A person in her twenties will have a slightly different to-do list than her fifty-something mother. As with all the recommendations made in this book, these are based on scientific research and follow generally accepted guidelines in the medical community.

20s

- ✓ **Blood Pressure:** Check this at least once a year or more frequently if it's previously been abnormally high or low.
- ✓ **Fasting Cholesterol:** Get your cholesterol tested after you have fasted for nine to twelve hours, which will give you a more accurate picture of your important lipid numbers: total cholesterol, LDL and HDL cholesterol, as well as triglyceride levels. You'll want to do this test every five years or more frequently if you've had an abnormal test result.
- ✓ **Dental Health:** Visit a dentist annually for a checkup and professional cleaning. Go twice a year if your mouth is prone to problems like tooth decay.
- ✓ **Eye Health:** Visit an ophthalmologist (eye doctor)

for an eye exam every two years or as your doctor recommends.

✓ **Sexual Health:** Get tested for sexually transmitted diseases; women should have an annual Pap smear and pelvic exam.

✓ **Immunizations:** Get a tetanus-diphtheria booster shot at age nineteen and the vaccine for human papillomavirus if you haven't already; get a flu vaccine every year. Individuals born in 1980 or later should receive a second varicella (chicken pox) vaccine.

✓ **Skin Exam:** Look for marks or changes on your skin monthly and have a doctor do an annual skin check.

✓ **Testicular Exam:** Perform a monthly self-exam, especially if there is a family history of testicular cancer.

✓ **Breast Exam:** Perform a monthly self-exam, especially if there is a family history of breast cancer.

✓ **Exercise:** Develop a personal exercise program and also keep track of your movement during the day with an accelerometer, and develop a daily personal activity target.

✓ **Diabetes Screening:** Have your hemoglobin A1c (also called glycosylated hemoglobin) checked if you have a family history of diabetes, a BMI greater than or equal to 25, or history of gestational diabetes. The hemoglobin A1c test will give you your average blood sugar value over the previous three months and is a better indicator of your overall number than a test that just looks at your blood-sugar value at a single moment in time.

30s

✓ **Blood Pressure:** Check this at least once a year or more frequently if it's previously been abnormally high or low.

✓ **Fasting Cholesterol:** Get your cholesterol tested every five years or more frequently if you've had an abnormal test result. A fasting cholesterol is taken after you've gone without eating for nine to twelve hours and gives a more accurate test result.

✓ **Dental Health:** Visit a dentist annually for a checkup and professional cleaning. Go twice a year if your mouth is prone to problems like tooth decay.

✓ **Eye Health:** Visit an ophthalmologist (eye doctor) for an eye exam every two years or as your doctor recommends.

✓ **Sexual Health:** Get tested for sexually transmitted diseases; women should have an annual Pap smear and pelvic exam.

✓ **Immunizations:** Maintain booster shots and get the annual flu vaccine.

✓ **Skin Exam:** Look for marks or changes on your skin monthly and have a doctor do an annual skin check.

✓ **Testicular Exam:** Perform a monthly self-exam, especially if there is a family history of testicular cancer.

✓ **Breast Exam:** Perform a monthly self-exam, especially if there is a family history of breast cancer.

✓ **Exercise:** Develop a personal exercise program and also keep track of your movement during the day with an accelerometer, and develop a daily personal activity target.

✓ **Diabetes Screening:** Have your hemoglobin A1c (also called glycosylated hemoglobin) checked if you have a family history of diabetes, a BMI greater than or equal to 25, or history of gestational diabetes. The hemoglobin A1c test will give you your average blood sugar value over the previous three months and is a better indicator of your overall number than a test that just looks at your blood-sugar value at a single moment in time.

40s

✓ **Blood Pressure:** At your doctor's office, check this at least once a year or more frequently if it's previously been abnormally high or low. At home, aim to keep tabs on your blood pressure more regularly and record your numbers. Notice any patterns that occur, such as your BP rising every afternoon or lowering after exercise.

✓ **Fasting Cholesterol and Inflammation Markers:** Get these tested every three to five years or more frequently if you've had an abnormal test result. Inflammation markers are compounds in the blood that reflect systemic inflammation going on in the body—signaling that something isn't right.

✓ **Dental Health:** Visit a dentist annually for a checkup and professional cleaning. Go twice a year if your mouth is prone to problems like tooth decay.

✓ **Eye Health:** Visit an ophthalmologist (eye doctor) for an eye exam every two years or as your doctor recommends.

✓ **Sexual Health:** Get tested for sexually transmitted diseases; women should have an annual Pap smear and pelvic exam.

✓ **Immunizations:** Maintain booster shots and get the annual flu vaccine.

✓ **Skin Exam:** Look for marks or changes on your skin monthly and have a doctor do an annual skin check.

✓ **Testicular Exam:** Perform a monthly self-exam, especially if there is a family history of testicular cancer.

✓ **Breast Exam:** Perform a monthly self-exam, especially if there is a family history of breast cancer; ask about when you should get your first mammogram. Annual mammography in this age group has been confirmed to decrease mortality but is not recommended by all professional organizations due to differing risk-benefit analyses. Options for breast cancer screening should be discussed with your provider yearly.

✓ **Exercise:** Develop a personal exercise program and also keep track of your movement during the day with an accelerometer, and develop a daily personal activity target.

✓ **Diabetes Screening:** Get your blood sugar tested at least once a year, more frequently if you've had an abnormal test result. Be sure to get your hemoglobin A1c test by age forty-five. This test will give you your average blood sugar value over the previous three months and is a better indicator of your overall number than a test that just looks at your blood-sugar value at a single moment in time.

✓ **Prostate Exam:** Get your baseline PSA test (an indicator for prostate cancer) if you're African American or there is a family history of prostate cancer; otherwise, you can wait until age fifty.

✓ **Preventive Medications:** Have the discussion with your doctor about whether a daily aspirin (75 or 81 milligrams) and statin make sense as preventive therapy based on your family history and personal risk factors.

50s

✓ **Blood Pressure:** At your doctor's office, check this at least once a year or more frequently if it's previously been abnormally high or low. At home, aim to keep tabs on your blood pressure more regularly and record your numbers. Notice any patterns that occur, such as your BP rising every afternoon or lowering after exercise.

✓ **Fasting Cholesterol and Inflammation Markers:** Check these every three to five years or more frequently if you've had an abnormal test result.

✓ **Colorectal Exam:** Get an annual fecal occult blood testing; and consider a colonoscopy every five to ten years depending on your doctor's recommendations based on your personal risks.

✓ **Dental Health:** Visit a dentist annually for a checkup and professional cleaning. Go twice a year if your mouth is prone to problems like tooth decay.

✓ **Diabetes Screening:** Get your blood sugar tested— including the hemoglobin A1c test—at least once a year, more frequently if you've had an abnormal test result.

✓ **Eye Health:** Visit an ophthalmologist (eye doctor) for an eye exam every two years or as your doctor recommends.

✓ **Immunizations:** Maintain booster shots and get the annual flu vaccine.

✓ **Osteoporosis Screening:** Get a bone density test if risk factors are present. Examples of risk factors include family history of the disease, taking steroids or other certain medications, going through menopause, sedentary lifestyle, excessive alcohol consumption, tobacco use, having an eating disorder, or having had weight loss surgery.

✓ **Prostate Exam:** Undergo a prostate exam annually that gives you PSA values, which are indicators of prostate cancer.

✓ **Skin Exam:** Look for marks or changes on your skin monthly and have a doctor do an annual skin check.

✓ **Breast Exam:** Perform a monthly self-exam, especially if there is a family history of breast cancer; schedule routine mammography based on your risk factors.

✓ **Exercise:** Develop a personal exercise program and also keep track of your movement during the day with an accelerometer, and develop a daily personal activity target.

✓ **Preventive Medications:** Have the discussion with your doctor about whether a daily aspirin (75 or 81 milligrams) and statin make sense as preventive therapy based on your family history and personal risk factors.

60s

✓ **Abdominal Ultrasound:** Have this test done if you're older than age sixty-five and have smoked.

✓ **Blood Pressure:** At your doctor's office, check this at least once a year or more frequently if it's previously been abnormally high or low. At home, aim to keep tabs on your blood pressure more regularly and record your numbers. Notice any patterns that occur, such as your BP rising every afternoon or lowering after exercise.

✓ **Fasting Cholesterol and Inflammation Markers:** Check these every five years or more frequently if you've had an abnormal test result.

✓ **Colorectal Exam:** Get a colorectal exam annually. This includes, until age seventy-five: colonoscopy every ten years; fecal occult blood testing every three years with sigmoidoscopy every five years; or annual fecal occult blood testing.

✓ **Dental Health:** Visit a dentist annually for a checkup and professional cleaning. Go twice a year if your mouth is prone to problems like tooth decay.

✓ **Diabetes Screening:** Check the A1c every three years or as your doctor recommends.

✓ **Eye Health:** Visit an ophthalmologist (eye doctor) for an eye exam every two years or as your doctor recommends.

✓ **Immunizations:** Maintain booster shots and get the annual flu vaccine; get the shingles/herpes zoster vaccine once after age sixty and pneumococcal vaccine (Pneumovax) at age sixty-five.

✓ **Hearing Test:** If you are over age sixty-five, have your hearing checked.

✓ **Osteoporosis Screening:** Get a bone density test if risk factors are present and at age sixty-five for all women.

✓ **Prostate Exam:** Undergo a prostate exam annually.

✓ **Breast Exam:** Perform a monthly self-exam, especially if there is a family history of breast cancer; schedule routine mammography based on your risk factors.

✓ **Skin Exam:** Look for marks or changes on your skin monthly and have a doctor do an annual skin check.

✓ **Exercise:** Develop a personal exercise program and also keep track of your movement during the day with an accelerometer, and develop a daily personal activity target.

✓ **Preventive Medications:** Have the discussion with your doctor about whether a daily aspirin (75 or 81 milligrams) and statin make sense as preventive therapy based on your family history and personal risk factors.

70s and Beyond

- ✓ **Abdominal Ultrasound:** Have this test done if you've smoked.
- ✓ **Blood Pressure:** At your doctor's office, check this at least once a year or more frequently if it's previously been abnormally high or low. At home, aim to keep tabs on your blood pressure more regularly and record your numbers. Notice any patterns that occur, such as your BP rising every afternoon or lowering after exercise.
- ✓ **Fasting Cholesterol and Inflammation Markers:** Check these every year or more frequently if you've had an abnormal test result.
- ✓ **Colorectal Exam:** Get an annual fecal occult blood testing; and consider a colonoscopy every five to ten years depending on your doctor's recommendations based on your personal risks.
- ✓ **Dental Health:** Visit a dentist annually for a checkup and professional cleaning. Go twice a year if your mouth is prone to problems like tooth decay.
- ✓ **Diabetes Screening:** Check the A1c every three years or as your doctor recommends.
- ✓ **Eye Health:** Visit an ophthalmologist (eye doctor) for an eye exam every two years or as your doctor recommends.
- ✓ **Immunizations:** Maintain booster shots and the annual flu vaccine; get the pneumococcal vaccine after age sixty-five if you didn't get it in your sixties.

✓ **Hearing Test:** If you are experiencing hearing loss, get your hearing checked.

✓ **Prostate Exam:** Undergo a prostate exam annually.

✓ **Breast Exam:** Perform a monthly self-exam, especially if there is a family history of breast cancer; schedule routine mammography based on your risk factors.

✓ **Skin Exam:** Look for marks or changes on your skin monthly and have a doctor do an annual skin check.

✓ **Exercise:** Develop a personal exercise program and also keep track of your movement during the day with an accelerometer, and develop a daily personal activity target.

✓ **Preventive Medications:** Have the discussion with your doctor about whether a daily aspirin (75 or 81 milligrams) and statin make sense as preventive therapy based on your family history and personal risk factors.

Health Lists

Below are some fun health lists I've put together and some that I've compiled from various readily available sources. They are the ultimate cheat sheet and will help you to remember key facts, rules, and ideas.

Regardless of age, the most important things you can do to stay healthy are:

✓ Have an annual physical exam. Find a doctor and make an appointment the same time every year for a general health check. Most people, especially if they are young and healthy, typically don't see a doctor for an annual check. Getting regular checks, preventative screening tests, and immunizations are among the most important things you can do to stay healthy. Take a personal health inventory questionnaire like the one available at my website (http://davidagus.com/hq) and bring the answers to your doctor's office.

✓ Know your family history. Family history is one of the most underused but extremely powerful tools for understanding your health. Family history affects your level of risk for cancer, diabetes, heart disease, and stroke, among other illnesses. It all starts with a conversation, so talk to your family members and keep a close eye out for any illnesses that a direct relative has experienced.

✓ Don't smoke. If you do smoke, stop! Compared to nonsmokers, men who smoke are about twenty-three times more likely to develop lung cancer. Smoking causes about 90 percent of lung cancer deaths and doubles your risk of heart disease.

✓ Be physically active. If you are not already physically active, start small and work up to a minimum of thirty minutes of moderate aerobic activity most days of the week. Also move during the day while at work and when you are engaged in other activities. Long periods of sitting raise the risk for disease. Everything counts—take the stairs instead of the

elevator, go for a twenty-minute walk during your
lunch break, and park on the far side of the lot at
the store.

✓ Keep it regular. As best you can, you should eat,
sleep, and exercise at the same time each day.

✓ Know your body. You should record every sign and
symptom you experience and discuss them with
your doctor.

✓ Eat a healthy diet. Fill up with fruits, vegetables, and
whole grains and choose healthy proteins like lean
meats, poultry, fish, beans, and nuts. Eat foods low
in processed fats, salt, and added sugars. Moderation
is key!

✓ Stay at a healthy weight. Balance calories from
foods and beverages with calories you burn off by
physical activity. Only 33 percent of adults are at a
healthy weight for their height. Obesity and being
overweight pose a major risk for chronic diseases,
including type-2 diabetes, cardiovascular disease,
hypertension, stroke, and certain cancers.

✓ Manage your stress. Stress, particularly long-term
stress, can be a factor in the onset or worsening of
ill health. Managing your stress is essential to your
health and well-being; take a timeout each day and
go for a walk or do something you find relaxing.

✓ Drink alcohol only in moderation. Alcohol can be
part of a healthy, balanced diet, but only if consumed
in moderation. This means no more than two drinks
a day for men, and one drink a day for women (a

standard drink is one 12-ounce bottle of beer or wine cooler, one 5-ounce glass of wine, or 1.5 ounces of 80-proof distilled spirits).

✓ Sleep well. The quality of your sleep can dictate how much you eat, how fast your metabolism runs, how fat or thin you are, how well you can fight off infections, and how well you can cope with stress. Keep a regular pattern of sleep; going to bed and waking up at roughly the same time is key.

✓ Avoid all vitamins and supplements. These should be avoided unless your physician tells you they are necessary.

✓ Discuss the role of aspirin and statins. Ask your doctor about using these preventive medications if you are forty or older.

Top 10 Actions to Reduce Your Risk for Illness

Taking these actions today can reduce your risk of becoming sick, especially for the two most dreaded diseases in later life: cancer and dementia.

1. Eat real food on a regular schedule.
2. Avoid vitamins and supplements.
3. Discuss aspirin and statins with your doctor when you are staring at age forty.
4. Follow the prescribed cancer screening schedules.
5. Exercise regularly and move during the day.
6. Maintain a healthy weight.
7. Avoid tobacco products.

8. Avoid direct sun exposure without sunscreen.
9. Avoid sources of inflammation.
10. Get a yearly flu shot.

Top 10 Things to Help Educate Kids About Health and Wellness

1. Explain why. All too often we just tell our children what to do without explaining the reasons. If you don't understand why, find out.
2. Watch the Jamie Oliver videos and TED Talk about children and nutrition. You can access Jamie's videos at http://www.youtube.com/user/JamieOliver.
3. Be a good example.
4. Encourage activity.
5. Teach them the importance of digital-free downtime.
6. Vaccines, vaccines, vaccines.
7. Take them food shopping and to the farmers market and engage them in the kitchen when you're cooking.
8. If there is an illness in the family, empower children to play a role. Put together a fund-raiser, educate others, or develop a plan for the child to help the affected person.
9. Prepare them for pediatrician visits by having them review themselves. Go head to toe and do an inventory to see if anything hurts or has changed. Encourage them to make a list of questions for their doctor.
10. Let them keep their list of medical data: weight and height over the years, immunization records, list of hospitalizations, etc. They will soon develop the

attitude that they do have a role in their health care. Allow them to have private time with their doctor.

Top 10 Causes of Death in the United States*

1. Heart disease: 597,689 deaths
2. Cancer: 574,743 deaths
3. Chronic lower respiratory diseases: 138,080 deaths
4. Stroke (cerebrovascular diseases): 129,476 deaths
5. Accidents (unintentional injuries): 120,859 deaths
6. Alzheimer's disease: 83,494 deaths
7. Diabetes: 69,071 deaths
8. Nephritis, nephrotic syndrome, and nephrosis: 50,476 deaths
9. Influenza and pneumonia: 50,097 deaths
10. Intentional self-harm (suicide): 38,364 deaths

Top 10 Causes of Death Worldwide**

1. Ischemic heart disease: 7.25 million deaths (12.8 percent of deaths)
2. Stroke and other cerebrovascular disease: 6.15 million deaths (10.8%)
3. Lower respiratory infections: 3.46 million deaths (6.1%)
4. Chronic obstructive pulmonary disease: 3.28 million deaths (5.8%)
5. Diarrheal diseases: 2.46 million deaths (4.3%)

---

* Data from the Centers for Disease Control and Prevention expressed as deaths in the United States for the 2010 calendar year.

** Data from the World Health Organization on worldwide deaths for the 2008 calendar year.

6. HIV/AIDS: 1.78 million deaths (3.1%)
7. Trachea, bronchus, and lung cancers: 1.39 million deaths (2.4%)
8. Tuberculosis: 1.34 million deaths (2.4%)
9. Diabetes mellitus: 1.26 million deaths (2.2%)
10. Road traffic accidents: 1.21 million deaths (2.1%)

Popular Weight Loss Myths*

- A little goes a long way. You can walk your way to weight loss. Truth: It takes effort to lose weight. You need more than a brisk walk a day to take—and keep—the weight off.
- Only realistic goals will help you to lose weight. Truth: You can set a preposterous goal and still make headway with weight loss.
- If you're overly ambitious with your weight loss efforts, you will fail. Truth: You can be as ambitious as you want despite the frustrations; it might keep you going.
- If you're not mentally ready to change your diet, you won't succeed. Truth: This is when just a little bit of motivation can really go a long way. If your mind is somewhat willing to make a few dietary shifts, you can succeed.
- If you lose weight fast, it won't last. Truth: Slow and steady doesn't always work. For some, fast weight loss can lead to lasting results.

---

* Source: http://www.nejm.org/doi/full/10.1056/NEJMsa1208051

Top 10 Foods High in Trans Fat*

1. Margarine, shortening, and other processed spreads
2. Packaged baking mixes (cake mixes, Bisquick)
3. Prepared soups (especially ramen noodles, soup cups)
4. Fast food (especially fried foods)
5. Frozen foods (products such as frozen pies, pot pies, waffles, pizzas, breaded fish sticks)
6. Baked goods (especially commercially baked products such as cakes and donuts)
7. Chips and crackers
8. Breakfast food (items like cereals and energy bars)
9. Cookies and candy (especially those that are cream filled)
10. Toppings and dips (products like nondairy creamers, flavored coffees, gravies, and salad dressings)

Top 10 Most Sugary Foods**

1. Granulated sugar and other sweeteners (brown sugar, honey, molasses, sorghum syrup)
2. Drink powders and soft drinks
3. Candies and nougat
4. Dried fruits
5. Cookies, cakes, and pies
6. Spreads, jams, and preserves
7. Cereals, cereal bars, and instant oatmeal packages
8. Sauces (products like ketchup, chocolate syrup, and salad dressing)

---

* Source: http://www.webmd.com/diet/features/
top-10-foods-with-trans-fats?page=3
** Source: http://www.healthaliciousness.com/articles/high-sugar-foods.php

9. Ice cream, milk shakes, café drinks
10. Canned fruit packed in syrup

Top High-Glycemic-Index Foods*

- Soft drinks, sports drinks, and fruit juices
- White bread, pasta, rice, and noodles (don't forget bagels, baguettes, donuts, waffles, pancakes, rice cakes, and pizza)
- Potatoes, potato chips, and parsnips
- Pretzels, commercial crackers, and cookies
- Cake and most baked goods
- Commercial cereals (refined) and instant oatmeal
- Dates, raisins, watermelon
- Most candy

Top 11 Fish with Omega-3**

1. Wild Alaskan Salmon
2. Arctic Char
3. Atlantic Mackerel
4. Pacific Sardines
5. Sablefish/Black Cod from Alaska or British Columbia
6. Anchovies
7. Oysters
8. Rainbow Trout

---

* Source: http://www.health.harvard.edu/newsweek/Glycemic_index_and_glycemic_load_for_100_foods.htm
** Source: US News and World Report summary from the Environmental Defense Fund's Seafood Selector and the Monterey Bay Aquarium's Seafood Watch programs (http://health.usnews.com/health-news/diet-fitness/slideshows/best-fish)

9. Albacore Tuna from the U.S. or Canada
10. Mussels
11. Pacific Halibut

Top 10 Fish with Mercury Contamination*

1. Tilefish (Gulf of Mexico)
2. Swordfish
3. Shark
4. King Mackerel
5. Bigeye Tuna
6. Orange Roughy
7. Marlin
8. Spanish Mackerel (Gulf of Mexico)
9. Grouper
10. Tuna

Top 10 Most Useful Health and Medicine Websites

(Note: this doesn't mean I agree with everything on the websites, just that they are a good sources of health information.)

1. National Institutes of Health (NIH.gov)
2. Centers for Disease Control and Prevention (CDC.gov)
3. American Academy of Family Physicians (familydoctor .org)
4. Office of Disease Prevention and Health Promotion (healthfinder.gov)

---

* Source: US FDA website data from commercial fish 1990–2010 (http:// www.fda.gov/Food/FoodborneIllnessContaminants/Metals/ucm115644 .htm).

  5. Livestrong (livestrong.org)
  6. American Heart Association (americanheart.org)
  7. The Mayo Clinic (MayoClinic.com)
  8. National Library of Medicine (MedlinePlus.gov)
  9. WebMD (WebMD.com)
10. American Cancer Society (cancer.org)

Top 5 Food Poisoning Culprits*

1. Poultry contaminated with *Campylobacter* or *Salmonella*
2. Beef and pork with the *Toxoplasma* parasite
3. Listeria in deli meats and dairy products like soft cheese
4. *Salmonella* and norovirus in multi-ingredient foods such as salads that are handled by food preparers (leafy greens are a leading source of food poisoning illnesses)
5. *Salmonella* in eggs and produce

Top 10 Reasons to Go to the ER**

  1. Difficulty breathing, shortness of breath
  2. Chest or upper abdominal pain or pressure
  3. Fainting, sudden dizziness, or weakness
  4. Changes in vision
  5. Confusion or changes in mental status
  6. Any sudden or severe pain
  7. Uncontrolled bleeding
  8. Severe or persistent vomiting or diarrhea
  9. Coughing or vomiting blood
10. Suicidal or homicidal feelings

---

* Source: Centers for Disease Control and Prevention
** Source: The American College of Emergency Physicians

Top 10 Things to Do During Cold Season

1. Get your flu shot if you haven't already.
2. Wash your hands routinely.
3. Avoid sharing food and drinks with others.
4. Stay away from sick people.
5. Don't go to work (and avoid public places) if you're feeling ill.
6. Keep zinc lozenges on hand.
7. Avoid touching your face and eating with your hands.
8. Carry hand sanitizer.
9. Avoid stuffy rooms that have poor ventilation.
10. Keep common surface areas clean.

Top 10 Reasons to Take a Walk

1. You'll prevent weight gain and perhaps walk off weight.
2. You'll reduce your risk of cancer.
3. You'll reduce your risk of heart disease and stroke.
4. You'll reduce your risk of diabetes.
5. You'll boost brain power and inspire creativity.
6. You'll improve your mood.
7. You'll relieve stress.
8. You'll stimulate a connection with nature and encourage self-reflection.
9. You'll gain an alertness on par with that you'd get from a cup of coffee.
10. You'll live longer.

Acknowledgments

As I did in my first book, I have my patients to thank, for they help me hone my message daily in my interactions with them. Thank you for allowing me to be involved with your care; you teach me daily about how the body works and remind me with every visit that my work isn't nearly complete. Medicine needs to be radically improved to assist and heal each of us. I also have to thank my critics, as their words and ideas inform my thinking and have helped me to further shape and clarify my message.

It is not just a privilege, but it is also a responsibility to educate about health. I have never been on this path alone and am indebted to many dedicated individuals. This book reflects the culmination of not just my lifetime work in the health-care industry, but also my ongoing collaboration with an expansive team. First, I have to thank my collaborator Kristin Loberg. Kristin and I have been working together for close to three years now, and when I considered putting another book together, I would have done it only with Kristin's involvement. She is an amazing partner, an insightful thinker, a remarkably talented writer, and a good friend.

I would like to thank her family, Lawrence and Colin (and baby number two, who is growing during the writing of this book), for allowing me to spend precious time with her over the past years. And I have to thank and applaud Chieun Ko, whose beautiful and sometimes cheeky illustrations both simplify the book's concepts and help make health fun. A big thanks to Chi's family, Brian and Luca, for sharing her with me over the past year.

Thanks to Robert Barnett, who has expertly and caringly represented, protected, and guided me through this process. David Povich, thank you for being my loving advocate and guardian. You have both been extraordinary in looking after me.

I have been with only one publishing house in my short career as an author, and I couldn't imagine a better and more supportive environment. I wish to thank my team at Simon & Schuster, led by Priscilla Painton, whose support, faith, and skill made this book possible. Her editorial insights and practical wisdom have helped me to create a much better book. Thanks also to her fantastic team, including Michael Accordino, Suzanne Donahue, Lance Fitzgerald, Larry Hughes, Nancy Inglis, Amy Ryan, Nancy Singer, Sydney Tanigawa, and the big chief, Jonathan Karp. Thank you for putting up with me and your continued support.

I am also indebted to my team at the USC Westside Cancer Center and the Center for Applied Molecular Medicine, who enables me to be both a physician and a researcher, and to find the time to write. I want to particularly thank my fantastic assistant, Autumn, and the clinic team of Adam, Angel, Claire, Julianne, Julie, Justine, Lisa, Olga, Robin, Shelly, and Mitchell. Thank you for your loyalty and friendship and the daily care you give to the patients we are honored to treat. To the research team of Jonathan, Parag, Dan, Shannon, Paul, Kian, Kristina, and Yvonne: thank you for pushing my thinking forward and dedicating yourself to figuring out better ways to treat disease.

I also have to thank those who continue to support and inspire me on a regular basis, including Jeff Fager, Sandy Gleysteen, Gayle King, Jonathan LaPook, Chris Licht, Norah O'Donnell, Karolyn Pearson, David Rhodes, and Charlie Rose at CBS News, who empower me to be able to educate and inform. To Dominick Anfuso, Marc Benioff, Gerald Breslauer, Eli Broad, Bill Campbell, Michael Dell, Larry Ellison, Robert Evans, Murray Gell-Mann, Al Gore, Brad Grey, Davis Guggenheim, Danny Hillis, Walter Isaacson, Peter Jacobs, Clifton Leaf, Max Nikias, Fabian Oberfeld, Howard Owens, Shimon Peres, Maury Povich, Carmen Puliafito, Bruce Ramer, Sumner Redstone, Joe Schoendorf, Dov Seidman, Bonnie Solow, Steven Spielberg, Elle Stephens, Yossi Vardi, Jay Walker, David Weissman, and Neil Young: your mentorship, friendship, and advice are truly appreciated.

Thanks to Steve Bennett and his team at AuthorBytes for their creative and dynamic website management, as well as Josh Greenstein, Amy Powell, and Karen Hermelin of Paramount Pictures for their fantastic guidance in getting people to listen to the "health" message.

Last, to my family, for their unwavering support and

love; thank you, Amy, Miles, Sydney, Mom, and Dad. For several generations now one of our family's best and most quoted traditions has been to always root for one another, and I couldn't have imagined a more heartfelt cheering section than the Povich and Agus extended families. Thank you all for your support, and for spreading my mission to better medicine and our health far and wide.

About the Author

Dr. David B. Agus is a professor of medicine and engineering at the University of Southern California Keck School of Medicine and Viterbi School of Engineering and heads USC's Westside Cancer Center and the Center for Applied Molecular Medicine. He is one of the world's leading cancer doctors, and the cofounder of two pioneering personalized medicine companies, Navigenics and Applied Proteomics. Dr. Agus is an international leader in new technologies and approaches for personalized health care and a contributor to CBS News. His first book, *The End of Illness*, became a *New York Times* #1 bestseller and was also the subject of a PBS special.